Weight Loss Zen

An Attitude Adjustment Guide
for Keto, Paleo & Low Carb Lifestyles

Dixie Vogel

Copyright

Printed in the United States of America
1st Printing: June, 2016

ISBN-13: 978-1533324009
ISBN-10: 153332400X

Low Carb Zen
2303 RR 620 S. #135-376
Lakeway, TX 78734

Book Updates & Freebies
www.lowcarbzen.com/zenbook

Dedication

This book is dedicated to everyone who has ever looked in the mirror and felt like a big, fat mess.

It's for everyone who has ever given up on a failed diet—and felt like giving up on themselves in the process.

It's for everyone who has ever broken down in tears or lost sleep over eating,

It's for everyone who has ever been scared of sitting down, unsure if the chair would hold up.

It's for everyone who has ever pretended not to care about weight but deep down, still really did.

It's for everyone who was just like me, fifteen years ago. This book is exactly what I would have told myself, had I had a clue.

This book is dedicated to you, courtesy of the countless folks who so generously shared their own journeys with me over the years. I am forever in their debt both on my own behalf, and on behalf of everyone with whom I've shared their wisdom.

Thank you for being here. Together, we've got this.

Contents

Attitude Adjustments..103

PREFACE

Journey Begins

"At your BMI, you have over a 45% chance of eventually developing diabetes."

My doctor looked sad as she handed me the graph, apparently resigned to her unenviable lot of providing vital information that will ultimately go unheeded.

I didn't have the mental facility just then to compare the scenario to Cassandra's curse via Apollo, forever more making accurate prophecies no one believed. I'm too much reeling from the smack in the face that word "diabetes" conjures up.

With the disease on both sides of my family (and abject terror at the thought of not being able to eat SUGAR, the horror!), I was dumbfounded. With my mouth being what it is, leaving me speechless is no small feat.

I'd already been very disturbed by a recent picture of me at the beach. And now, this. I did exactly what I would have advised friends or my kids to do in the same circumstance: I decided then and there to suck it up and make some serious changes.

Researching, I soon realized the people that had the most to lose (i.e. 100 pounds or more, like me) seemed to do best on low carb. The before and after pictures made a solid case. Atkins was the gold standard of low carb, so Atkins, here I come! And that was the not-so-glamorous beginning of what ultimately became my love affair with low carb.

A few months in, everybody in my life was sick of hearing about my diet and I wanted more support. So I joined an online community. As I became more knowledgeable and successful (losing well over 100 pounds), I was invited to become a moderator; I eventually bought the site and ran it another couple years. A series of personal circumstances led me to leaving that role, selling the site and slowly, gradually, almost imperceptibly, losing my way as well. Without the ongoing immersion in all things low carb, my habits just got sloppier and sloppier.

I put back on some of the weight, not because it was so impossible to maintain, but because I didn't stay focused. I'm aging and my body doesn't work the same as it used to. It becomes more difficult when you get older and especially if you don't always walk the straight and narrow.

I always will be what I call a "true believer" in the lifestyle, but I've lived in varying degrees of compliance. It's a lot of stress and responsibility to head up a weight loss community. I really didn't want to be forever looked to as an example (as you will, even without touting yourself as such). Because plenty of times, I would have been an awful example! Depending on what day you catch me, that's sometimes still true.

However, I kept my Low Carb page on Facebook up and running as a public service—I couldn't bear to delete its massive-to-me following of three thousand some fans.

But I was only thinking of low carb every now and then...until the page vent viral. Thanks to the help of my talented friends who were managing it, D.J. Foodie (of DJFoodie.com) and Theresa Marie (of LowCarbReviews.com), suddenly thousands of people were showing up every day, and it seemed like all of them had questions!

So I did the right thing when you're gifted an opportunity to make a difference: brushed up my skills and dove back in to the world of low carb recipes, science, and even controversy. It was either that, or let all these people down! I know low carb saves lives and here I was, in the position do that. How could I ignore the opportunity? I had long stopped seeking this role, but it was following me.

The Universe had spoken, and it said "low carb." (Find us at www.facebook.com/LowCarbZen.)

It's different for me, now. The losses are not as effortless as they were, years ago. Each time you slack and come back, it goes a little slower. Age and hormones and thyroid functioning all impact my personal journey. I don't feel like a failure because of that.

Instead, I ask myself the very same question I sometimes ask you: If you knew you'd never lose another pound, would you still follow this lifestyle?

That answer, for me, is simple and loud YES! I feel great. I know I'm taking care of my body. While many of us would love to lose weight, if you're doing this right, it's not JUST about weight. It's about living a healthy lifestyle, feeling good, and being kind to your body. That's one irony of weight loss Zen: not fixating on the losses helps you lose.

It's not always a straight line, from where you start to where you're going. However, I have discovered the better I treat my body, the better it treats me.

That's why I'm here. But what about you?

In truth, it doesn't matter if you're eating this way to lose weight or not. Many of the skills, attitudes and choices that come into play for weight loss are just as important for those following any special diet. Many are applicable to other areas of life as well. Sanity is sanity.

Heck, it doesn't really matter what you weigh at all! You realize that, right? If I could communicate only that one thought, I've been successful. It's true, health or aesthetics may initially lead us down this path. Or we may just feel better eating this way. But if you go through the rest of your life thinking still thinking it's all about the weight, you've missed the entire point!

You're not a better person if you're skinny than if you are fat. You're not worthy when you eat well and worthless when you don't. You're just as wonderful no matter your diet (or not, I don't know you).

Here's the thing: certain choices tend to support long-term goals like losing weight and improving health, while other approaches tend to sabotage those same goals. If you want to maximize your success reaching your OWN GOALS, I hope to offer some thoughts, insights and smart-ass remarks to help you do that. Fair enough?

Your value is not correlated with your pants size. It comes from within, Sparky. Always has, always will. Everything else is just window dressing.

Know that always, and value yourself.

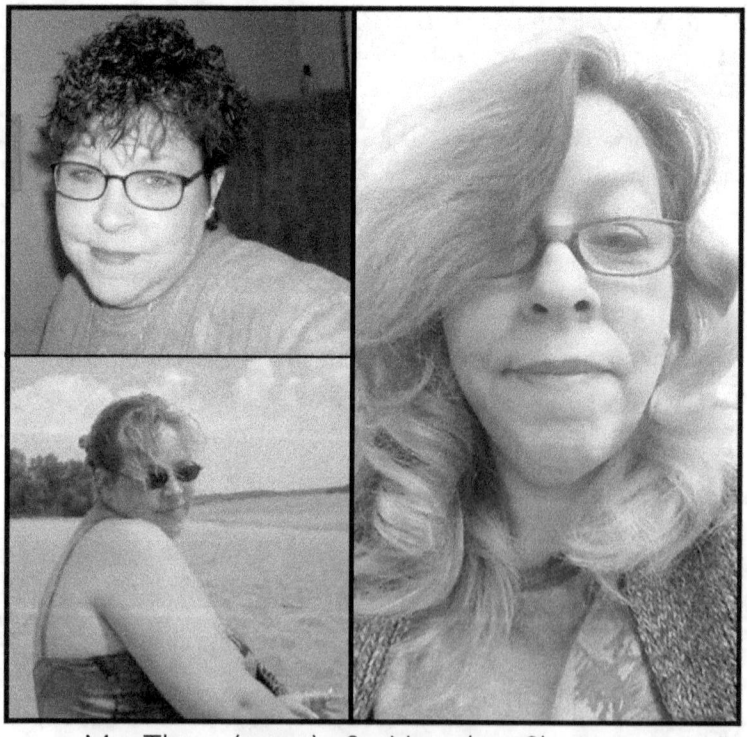

Me, Then (2003) & Now (2016)

INTRODUCTION

Too Fat to Be a Dieting Guru?

When I told my husband I was going to start making videos for my popular weight loss Facebook page, he looked utterly horrified.

I didn't get it.

"What? It's not like I'm going to hand out directions to our house or something."

I was confused. He's extremely supportive of my work. So it wasn't embarrassment.

But the look on his face suggested he thought I was undertaking something very, very dangerous.

"It's the Internet," he says, after a pause. "People are mean."

He was worried about my feelings! The man loves me. It's a beautiful thing.

Naturally, on the very first video I shared, someone commented that I was "way too fat" to be talking to people about weight loss. Her exact words were that I was "not a good advertisement."

Of course, I'm not a walking, talking advertisement! I'm a human being, with all the messiness, fallibility and general complications that condition entails.

Now, I knew it was coming, so it didn't throw me for a loop. The truth of the matter is, I'm EXACTLY the right person to talk to you about weight loss.

No, I'm not a doctor or a nurse. I'm not a scientist or a nutritionist or a personal trainer. I'm not a health food freak, or even a great cook. And I'm not your therapist, your priest or your mother.

I am, however, a chick who knows a lot about being overweight—including the real life struggles of everyday people who are overweight. I have spent the majority of my life in a condition doctors would classify as "morbidly obese."

I know what it's like to be fat. And it know what it's like to lose a lot of fat. And I pretty much know what it's like, every little bit in between.

I've led weight loss communities for years now, and during that time, have had the benefit of observing literally millions of people undertaking similar weight loss endeavors. Millions! It's mind blowing.

In that time, I've come to notice what sorts of attitudes, perspectives and approaches are very common to the people who do well, versus those common to those who struggle. And I've lived it.

Weight loss is a lot like sex: the most important bits happen in your head. I want to help you flip some switches in your head, to move from wherever you are right now, whatever struggles and frustrations you have with your own weight loss journey, to Zen.

The coolest part about finding Zen is that it makes your efforts so much more effective! And it enhances every other area of your life at the same time. It's win-win on steroids, man.

What I call "Weight Loss Zen" is about being in your groove, the place where you really hit your stride and what you're doing stops being a struggle.

It's when the whole enterprise stops being about rules, stops being about "no" and starts just being how you live.

It's the difference between what you "can't" have and what you can!

It's freedom from beating up on yourself and learning to honor your spirit and body while making solid decisions that support long term goals.

For many, Zen's nothing short of ending the tyranny a lying hunk of metal and gears (a.k.a. the scale) has long held over mood and sense of self-worth.

True Weight Loss Zen a gift I cannot give to you directly, but I can help you find it if you're seeking.

I've been blessed walk this path alongside some incredibly wise people and in those travels, I've picked up many useful tricks and tips, which I'm going to share with you.

Your job is to hear me out. That's it. Hear me out, consider what I have to say, and look at adopting what resonates with you.

I won't claim to know what works for everybody (or every single body), every time. Because this journey is as unique as each individual that undertakes it.

But I do understand a lot of what goes through the head of someone on this journey, both because of the multitudes I've interacted with on this path but much more intimately, because I'm on this path.

So if it sounds like I'm listening in to your brain in places, it's because I sort of am. But I'm probably much nicer to you than you are. So maybe that helps.

Enjoy the ride. We are so often all about the destination here. But most of our days are spent in the journey itself, after all. So we'd best make the most of it.

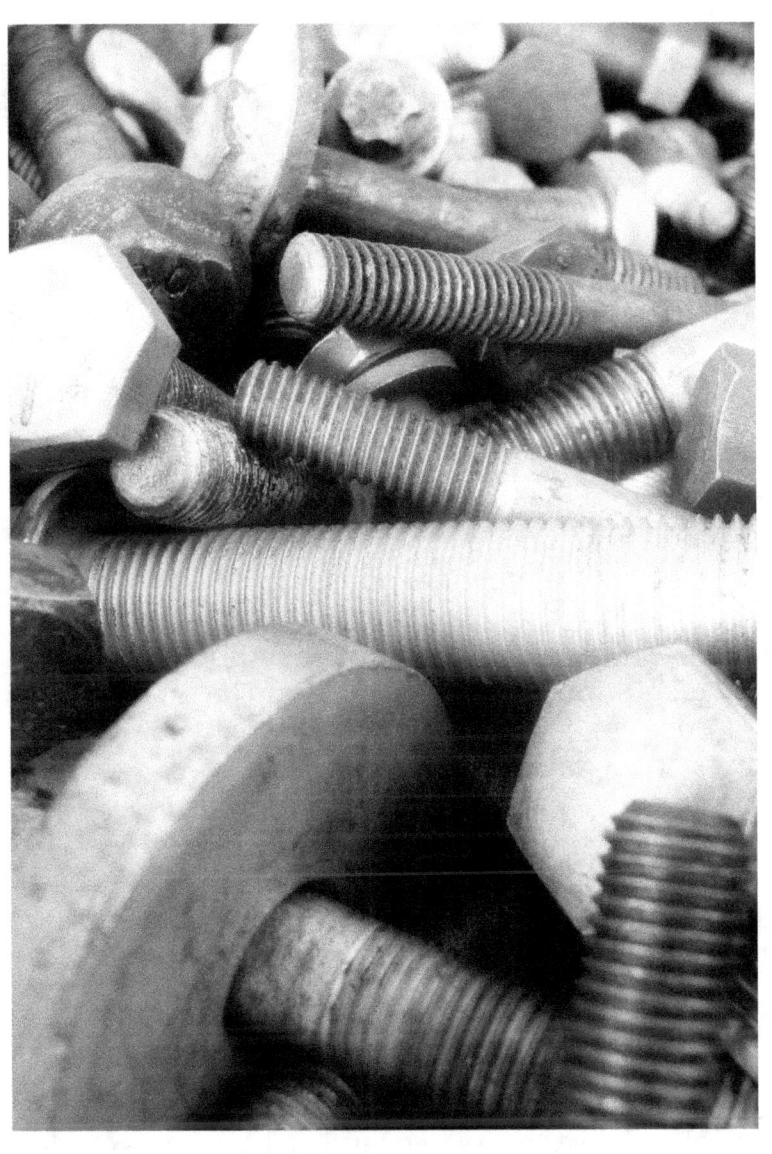

Noobs: Getting Started

CHAPTER 1

Resolving to Get it Right: Helpful Resolutions

Being involved in weight loss community for years, I've had opportunity to see lots of resolutions from dieters getting started.

Some resolutions help, while others clearly don't. Follow these tips to make yourself uplifting, helpful resolutions that you feel good about keeping.

Think behavioral resolutions as opposed to lose-by resolutions. That's because you have full control of behavior, but no control over what you may lose by what date. Our bodies are very complex organisms, and there is just an infinite number of variables that impact what poundage the body releases and when. Behavioral resolutions allow you to feel successful, which is vital to staying on course, and ultimately have the same payout on reaching weight loss goals if chosen wisely.

Ramp your way up, for goodness sakes! I cringe when I see someone who's been inactive for ages resolve to exercise two and a half hours a day, every day. This doesn't last because it's too much of a change, and the demands of making it all at once are just not sustainable. I know the intentions are good, but that's setting yourself up to fail while making the process much more painful. Give yourself breathing room. Give yourself a transitional period. Don't make the work of being kind to your body turn punitive. Make changes as pleasant as possible. You're much more likely to follow through long term that way.

Focus on the positive. Saying "I will not eat sugary cookies anymore" doesn't feel nearly as good as saying, "I'll create healthier versions of the cookies I love." Both statements have the same net worth. But the second statement isn't about restriction; it's about benefit! Benefit takes you much further.

Resolve to replace what you must leave behind. Use this same technique for any behavior you would like to eliminate. Find something that fulfills the need you're addressing with the old behavior. If you frequently eat to relax, resolve to give yourself regular time to read, listen to music, play a game or do something else you find relaxing instead. Address needs in more adaptive ways and you won't be swimming against the tide to stay focused.

Be playful. Resolutions don't have to be cranky, serious edicts based on "our own good." You can get the same benefits in more fun ways with some creativity. How about resolving to take a walk at sunset a few nights a week? Resolve to remind yourself before bedtime of something you feel good about from the day. Or resolve to spend more time playing with your pets. Resolve to trick a carb-lover into enjoying a low carb recipe! Make your resolutions rewarding and fun. You'll be more likely to follow through.

Resolve to forgive yourself. Forgive, both for slips and especially past behavior. If you're refocusing, great! Stop griping about where you are now, and start congratulating yourself for taking better care of yourself right now! You don't enjoy whining anyway, right? Self-recrimination is nothing but depressing. Depression is way fattening! People who feel good about themselves make better choices (and feel better doing it).

Resolve to pay attention. This is a very individual journey. What works for your friend will not always work for you. Consider this journey an advanced level course in how your body works, where the dividends for graduation will be paid in success.

Resolve to make change easier. Planning ahead, using all the resources at your disposal, and doing everything you can to make your life easier in any way whatsoever will actually make your path to weight loss smoother as well. A happy, relaxed dieter is most likely a successful dieter. Use your energy wisely.

Resolve to acknowledge and celebrate ALL successes, large and small. Nothing motivates like success, and yet so many people focus only on where they fall short in an effort to drive success. Bad idea. Success attracts more of the same.

Resolve to encourage others. One of the reasons weight loss communities flourish is because they work. Actively encouraging others isn't only the nice thing to do: it helps YOU do better following your own plan because you're focusing on healthy, adaptive behaviors. As a perk, you're also in good shape karmically and you're making the world a better place. (Gosh, I just love win-win!)

A Simple Test for Resolutions: does it further your goals AND feel good to practice? That's it. If you can answer "yes" to both these questions, you're on your way to achieving your goals because there is nothing that can keep you from soaring...

Not even you.

CHAPTER 2

Preparing to Get Busy

You've been thinking about it. And thinking about it. And thinking about it some more. You've mulled it, researched it, considered it, studied it and dissected it.

And you've decided. You're ready to drop the flab.

I know it can be challenging because more than anything else, much more than changing how you eat or live, this decision entails changing how you think, and how you've probably been thinking for years now!

So with that in mind, here are some of my best get-going tips, straight from the heart but shot from the hip.

Don't wait for the perfect time to get busy. Guess what, girlfriend(/boyfriend)? There AIN'T a perfect time, at least in the sense that everything is stress-free and there are no distractions and yada, yada, yada. Now is the only point in time where you have any power. So the only perfect time is NOW!

Stop worrying about the HOW. Frankly, life can provide us with a million and two avenues for success we would have never imagined on our own. If you have to figure out exactly how it's gonna happen minute-by-minute before you start, you are drawing a box around the situation and adding inherent limits in forcing that level of definition. Life is a wonderful adventure, full of surprises of all sorts, and most of the greatest things that have happened to me were things I couldn't possibly have known to plan.

You must remain flexible and open to learning along the way. Just decide the what, and the how will take care of itself organically. This is hard to do at first because it involves a certain level of trust, but trust me: it works!

Let go of the WHEN, too! I mean, heck, how much does the when really matter anywho? People get ridiculously impatient to finish their weight loss project and be done with it. And while I understand this, changes take time and energy. You didn't get where you are overnight, so you won't get somewhere new overnight, either...and in this context, I'm talking about the "when is this going to be complete?" question. There is the other when, when to start. And that's now!

Stop worrying about what you "should" do first. You know what? It doesn't freakin' matter what you do first, or whether it seems like a big step or a small step or what. Just do something! Every step, however modest, takes you closer to your goals. Just do something today! Break it down and take one tiny piece of the puzzle and put it into place.

Let go of the whole "wasted time" concept. As in, "Well, I wasted all this time and if I'd done this two years ago, I'd be done." I mean, c'mon! If you got something out of it, learned something, grew somehow, then it's not wasted! And if you didn't, then take another look! 'Cause there's always something you can take from any experience.

It's not only counter-productive to define your time as wasted, it's just not fair to be angry with yourself for not being born fully evolved. If you're not happy with where you're at now, well, great, good that you can see it. Time to move on! But that doesn't mean that you haven't been exactly where you needed to be until now, either. This is a good thing, friend! I see the whole being ready to move on as evidence that you are growing and changing, and therefore doing EXACTLY what you need to be doing.

Listen to the messages. Now, I don't know what your spiritual beliefs are, and I don't care. But for me, I know that when I need to do something, I get messages of sorts. You can believe it's from spirit or you can believe it's my subconscious mind or you can believe I'm a lunatic. Your preference! But if you're open to this idea at all...once you start to pay attention, you'll hear a lot more messages. You'll see them in interactions and in things you hear on the radio and in magazine headlines or books or all over, clues that sort of jump out at you wherever you look.

The point is that when it's time to do something, just get off your butt and go, and you will feel it in your gut. You'll know it's right. You'll find the topic coming up again and again and you'll be more attuned to circumstances and facts surrounding what you need to do. People make the mistake of ignoring their intuition, talking themselves out of their own, preciously valuable insights all the time. Your intuition is your best friend! Use it to your advantage and you'll be amazed at how things start to magically "fall together" for you.

Appreciate progress from every single step you take, however insignificant you may believe that step to be. When you take time out to feel good about what you're doing and the progress that you're making, it's motivating. You're generating good energy for yourself, which builds more energy and momentum. It works for you just like it works for others: appreciation for efforts leads to greater efforts. Who works harder at a job: the person who feels like efforts are unnoticed and minimized, or the person who feels like contributions are valued? You are your body's boss. Be a kind, encouraging boss!

Remember, folks: this is a chain reaction. One step leads to another, which leads to another. Every step counts because every step is connected in the chain from where you're at now to where you're going.

Consider any setbacks you encounter education. It's all prep work for getting to where you're going, man. Every little snag, you can learn something. Every minor delay, you can use to your advantage. Setbacks only become failures if you let them conquer you instead of using them for what they really are: a source of vital information about moving ahead, circumventing troubles and pitfalls. Not to mention your experiences of setback may be helpful to others, if you choose to share.

Focus on the right stuff. Don't focus on losing X number of pounds. Focus on what losing the weight will actually DO for you. It's not a magic number on the scale; it's the health or energy or confidence level that goes along with it, you know? When you do this, you open yourself to as many potential avenues for progress as possible, many of which will support your weight loss efforts even if they have nothing whatsoever to do with weight loss. Sometimes people lose sight of their own hard-earned successes because they will be distracted by whatever measure of progress they've fixated on (read: scale numbers) instead of the outcome they were actually seeking (like health or energy).

And speaking of flexibility: be flexible! Conditions change as you go and if you're paying attention, you will be learning plenty along the trip. So incorporate it all into your journey! It's great to have a roadmap to get started, but remain open to little detours and alterations as you live and learn along the trip. You may well be surprised at what you find when you follow your instincts and stay open to the gifts that are out there.

Let go of the fear, because it's not rational (and most feared outcomes, like failure, are usually not as bad as doing nothing anyway). If it doesn't work out the way you want, you may feel sad or upset about not reaching your initial goal. Okay. But if you have made improvements and are learning, you're already much better off than when you started regardless. You can paralyze yourself with terror of failure, but to what ends? You end up guaranteeing failure by being afraid to start, so it becomes a self-fulfilling prophecy.

Continually work on making the necessary mental adjustments. I am a firm believer that every change you make on the outside starts on the inside. If your brain isn't prepped to accept and accommodate the change, it just won't work long term for you. You can have all the conditions primed and the tools at the ready and even be doing the stuff you need to do, but if your mind hasn't accepted it, whatever progress you make just won't stick for good.

This is where visualization comes in handy. If you keep visualizing, you are training your brain to accept the vision of your desired outcome as reality. Science has found the body actually has some difficulty distinguishing between real experiences and vividly imagined experiences (although I don't recommend merely imagining you're eating right and calling it done.) I don't think anybody completely understands the mind-body connection and all the implications, but you'd have to be clueless to claim there isn't a connection.

Mostly though, just DO. Whatever comes to your mind, whatever feels right, whatever seems the easiest way to start, it doesn't matter a whit. Just start! Any action you take towards your goals will help you feel stronger and more in control. All progress counts! We're talking the turtle and the hare, here. It's not the huge strides or the lightening fast motion that gets you there; it's the little steps, day in and day out, the modest but consistent progress.

Never focus on how far you have to go. Always look at how far you've come! If you are focusing on how far you have to go, how much there is to do, I can promise, you're gonna feel overwhelmed. But if you keep yourself attuned to progress and the many successes on the journey, you'll want to build more of 'em. This isn't to say you shouldn't daydream about where you're going, either. Honestly, I think that's productive for helping your brain switch gears and maintain your success overall. But if the focus starts shifting from a pleasant, light, happy thing to a burdensome, ominous, how-far-I-still-have-to-go thing, you need to switch it around.

When in doubt about which option to take, always choose what gives the most joy. You can tell me sugar brings you joy, but if it makes you sick long term, that's not joy. That's addiction. Life is to be lived. It's about love and joy and happiness and contentment. I know sometimes there are lots of considerations, but long-term joy orientation has absolutely never steered me wrong. The more we can bring our lives into tune with who we are inside, the more joy we feel and the better off we'll be.

Know thyself and act accordingly. Do whatever you're doing in a way you're comfortable with, because you will naturally have a sense of the approach that fits your personality best. When we start on a big journey, we're going to experience a certain level of discomfort because of making big changes. I'm talking about a deeper level here, finding ways to go forward that fit in with who you really are. Recognize how your goals fit with your personal approach to life.

If you're most comfortable with a very tick-tock, quantified, measured sort of reality, then absolutely, approach the situation from that angle and find ways to tick-tock your path. You may find detailed meal plans, lots of tracking and scheduled eating times work great for you. The detail-oriented macro breakdown of Ketogenic eating may fit your personality like a glove.

If you're a rule-hating free spirit (like me), then find ways to approach your path that fit a rule-hating personality. Keto percentage tracking would drive me insane, so I don't do Keto. Eating simply like our Paleo friends do, keeping loose tabs on how many carbs I'm eating and paying mind to hunger levels works well for me. I'm all about being in tune with my body and energy levels.

But whatever you do, you MUST turn this journey into your own. There are many paths to the same destination. Take the path that bests accommodate who YOU are. See, you've got the best shot for lasting change if you merge what you're doing with who you really are. The more authentically your changes reflect your personal reality, the more likely they are going to be permanent. And that's what we're shooting for.

Most of all, smell the flowers. We can sometimes get caught up in all the fervor and swirling winds that come with big changes, and forget why we're doing what we're doing to begin with. Life is NOT a destination, but a journey. Look for the beauty in your journey. It's everywhere, if you are willing to open yourself up to it. Keep laughing, keep looking for the flowers along the way. You'll find them in the most unlikely places, sometimes.

Don't wait for your life to start, 'cause I got a news flash: it's here, baby! You're knee-deep in your life right this second, man! So take a deeeeeep breath, look around you, and soak up that experience. This is what gives you focus. Feel the beauty, appreciating the good surrounding you. If you spend a few minutes of every single day noticing all that is wondrous and beautiful and just feeling gratitude for it, I can tell you this: you will get your energy and focus recharged exponentially. It's palpable.

I know a lot of people approach weight loss (and maybe change in general) from a place of deficiency and a sense of inadequacy, but I believe that's completely unnecessary and complicates the process. In fact, it's more than unnecessary. It's counterproductive and hurtful. So stop it!

The fact you're not feeling satisfied with the status quo is a very good thing; it says you're growing and ready to move on. Awesome!

But no need to feel bad. You choose the status quo either directly or by default, so it undoubtedly served you in some way at some point, fulfilled some need in your life. Maybe you needed to feel pleasure, comforted or safe. Maybe you needed a way to manage stress. Maybe you needed to understand the importance of taking care of your body. Whatever the old way of eating and living did for you, it undoubtedly provided something. Even if that something ultimately is to stress how important taking good care of yourself is now.

So don't curse the past you. That's not fair. Thank the past you, for doing what was needed for you at the time.

But now your needs are different now and you're ready to move on and evolve a little bit.

So let's get busy evolving!

CHAPTER 3

10 Easy Steps to Actually Starting

Having trouble knowing where to start? Know that you need to lose weight, you want to lose weight, you are committed to losing weight, but you're maybe feeling a bit lost as to knowing exactly what to do to start?

Well, I've got you covered with getting started advice!

Start reading up on plans to decide which one is best-suited for your lifestyle. Learn how and why your plan works, so when your mother worries about you "losing too much weight" or friends chide you for "not eating healthy," you're confident. Get informed!

Read success stories, any place you can find them. Look at LOTS of before/after pictures. This will help you start to believe it's possible for YOU. Once you start believing, you're on your way.

In the meantime, begin clearing your home of the most difficult off-plan foods. While your family may whimper for a few days, you're not only helping yourself by doing this. You're giving them a wonderful gift as well: better health for the entire family! They will get over it. And if they don't, you have more serious issues to address than your eating habits. Not to be snippy, but you know. It's your health we're talking here.

Work on improving eating behaviors and activity levels. Eat more veggies, less sugar and processed foods, drink more water, and move around just a bit more. Whatever you can start with that's not too painful for you, do it now!

Go shopping. Have pre-made snacks on hand for when you're hungry. There is no reason to struggle with temptation when you can plan instead. Planning trumps willpower every single time.

Visualize success. SEE yourself as successful, imagine it, feel it, and start defining yourself as successful—not for reaching a particular goal, but for making vital progress in taking care of yourself. That is a success you can claim immediately, and it will help you get started on building a long-running string of successes.

DO IT! All the thinking about it, talking about it, reading about it, contemplating it, analyzing it, debating it or dreaming about it does nothing if you don't just DO it. There is no right time other than NOW. You don't have to be perfect, you don't have to know everything, and you don't have to be without error. You just have to keep going. If you slip, keep going. Just keep going, keep doing it no matter what.

That is the biggest secret to success, you know: KEEP GOING! Let go of the "how will it work" bit—

really just a veiled excuse to avoid action, insisting on seeing every step of the process in your head before beginning—and move on to merely, mindfully doing. You take care of today, every day, and results take care of themselves.

Stop counting the minutes! Don't try to figure out your end date, because if you want this to work for you permanently, you have to incorporate how you eat into your daily lifestyle, permanently. Toss that calendar out the window! Don't compare yourself to others, don't weigh yourself seven times a day, don't set hard and fast (and arbitrary) must-lose-by dates. That's all counterproductive.

Focusing on speed does two things: 1.) Making yourself feel like a failure when one of those best-case-scenario, arbitrary time goals doesn't pan out; and 2.) Reinforcing the "crash-diet-lose-the-weight-super-fast-and-then-go-back-to-eating-normally" mentality. If you go back to eating like you used to, you'll go back to weighing what you used to. You're not on a diet, you're changing how you eat for-ev-er.

Ignore setbacks and remain singularly focused on progress and the process. We sometimes use setbacks as excuses to feel bad and hop off the wagon into a big vat of cookie dough. Setbacks, slipups, or "cheats" (although I don't personally care for that word) mean exactly what you DECIDE they mean and nothing more. They can spiral you into days, weeks or months of off-plan eating if you interpret them as a failure—giving yourself even more to recover from (and eating mid guilt-fest isn't very satisfying, anyway)—or setbacks can help you learn your own body better, coming to know your own rhythms and what tends to lead you off-course. You can decide if it's a help or hindrance to you. There are no real mistakes: only learning experiences.

Throughout, focus on what you're getting, not what you're giving up. You'll find shortly that you're not really giving up anything worthwhile anyway. There is no "can't." You CAN eat anything you want. You can also stay fat or unhealthy. But it's your choice, always. The fact of the matter is that you get what you focus on. If you focus on the sugar-loaded garbage you think you're missing out on, you'll end up eating that. If not now, eventually. If you focus on the fabulous and healthy new you, well, you'll get that, too.

Truth is, it's easier than you think it will be. The anticipation is far worse than the actual event, really. Once you get started (and get past the initial discomfort of changing your habits), you will find it's not all that tough, and it's SO worth it! I swear it is.

So let's get cooking already!

CHAPTER 4

Eating Plan Prep: Planning for Success

The little things do add up! When you're preparing to take the new diet plunge, here is exactly how to get ready.

First off, you need to pick a plan and get the book for your plan. This is vital, because it gives you a roadmap to success, and it DOES make a huge difference. Many of the folks I know are on Atkins (so "the book" for that is *A New Atkins for a New You*), but whichever plan you pick is fine. The important part is that you DO select a plan, and you do get the corresponding book. Let's add it up: how well has "your way" been working for you thus far? Yeah. 'Nuff said, huh? Be sure to give your plan at least two full weeks to start as a commitment, following it explicitly and see where it takes you.

I like to point out that I've done low-carb twice. The first time, I heard about the plan and tried to follow it based on what other people said. I lasted two weeks and lost 12 pounds. Not bad, except...the next time, I got the book and did my homework. That was November 2003, and I'm still low-carbing. I've lost over 100 pounds and I feel great. Which results would you prefer?

[Aside: Please don't say you just can't afford to get the book. You can't afford NOT to get the book. A paperback, used or Kindle copy of a diet plan book costs somewhere around seven bucks. That's ONE trip to McDonalds, a couple of Starbucks Lattés, less than a single lunch out. Not to mention that wonderful institution we call the Library. Except to be frank, if you're not willing to invest $7 in the rest of your life, there isn't much I can say that will be of help to you. Get the %(^*% book already!]

In the meantime, start cutting back on that sugar consumption. You don't have to quit at first, but cut down as much as you feel comfortable doing right now. Slow down on white flour products and processed foods as well, and replace some of your liquid consumption with water.

I recommend drinking 1/2 your body weight in oz. of water daily, long term. It takes a while to work up to this level, but it is a huge help! Start eating more veggies. Pay attention to what's going into your mouth! Move around a bit; take a short walk after dinner. Whatever. Just start taking SMALL steps and moving in the direction you want to go.

What you're doing here is changing your HABITS from the ones that are keeping you overweight to ones that will help you be healthy for life. It doesn't have to be hard. In fact, those small changes that aren't hard are the best, because they are the least painful and you can start feeling a sense of success right away. Then build on them!

Start working on developing a slew of (non-eating) options for dealing with stress. Some ideas: journaling, taking a walk, baths, calling a friend, knitting, watching a movie, meditating, listening to music, whatever it is that flips your switch. Just have a list of things you can turn to when stress hits that are NOT related to eating.

And while we're at it, start getting rid of the crap in your fridge and cupboard! (I shouldn't have to say this, but I will: please don't "get rid of it" by shoving it down your piehole in one last blitz.) You don't need it there. It's so much easier to stay on track when temptations aren't readily available. And please don't tell me other folks in your home "need" those unhealthy foods: they need YOU much more!

Keep working on feeling good about you! Define yourself as a strong person who is ready, willing, and capable of moving forward. Use your language to reinforce that perception, even if you don't quite believe it yet. Your subconscious hears what you are saying and it begins to act accordingly. The evolution starts.

The know-how comes from reading your plan and researching; the drive comes from believing you can do it and getting a little success under your belt. Nothing motivates like success! Feeling good about yourself will help you keep going when it gets tough, as it sometimes does.

Yes, it absolutely takes more time and effort to plan first. A healthy plan, with lots of options ready to go, will always demand more of you than gliding along with your old, comfortable habits, effectively hitting the snooze button on your life.

I get that, because I have been sitting in your seat, debating whether to stop and get some meat and salad fixings at the grocery store or just drive through the local fast food joint, you know. Just this once. Because I'm tired.

I've done the "maybe someday" scenario for years at a time. Some folks? They never leave that place. But that fate doesn't need to be yours.

And once I started planning and following through on those plans, I found myself asking over and over again, "Why didn't I do this sooner?!"

One thing I promise you without reservation: it's WAY worth every bit of planning effort you put into it!

So here's to planning for success.

CHAPTER 5

Top 10 Rules for Losing it for Good

It's not a destination, but a process. All about the journey, as I'm fond of saying. Keep your attitude in check, and the rest falls into place. Here's my "Top 10" to keep you grounded.

There is NO failure. To fail is to quit. As long as you're moving, you are a success. Former attempts at weight loss? That was just practice! You're a masterpiece in progress.

Eating is NOT a moral issue. You are not a bad person based on what you eat, nor are you a good person based on what you haven't eaten. Yes, I love being thinner. I'm healthier and happier. But the truth is always the same: my value and self-worth are not determined by my dinner.

It's all about choice. You can eat whatever you want. The rub, of course, is in the consequences. Single choices are largely unimportant, but the choices you make most often come home to roost.

Ask yourself if a given choice ultimately supports your goals. And if you've made a choice that doesn't move you forward, fine. Just use it to learn instead of as an excuse to stay off-track. There are no mistakes!

Every single, tiny step counts. Every single effort matters. Take the stairs instead of the elevator? Walk around the block twice? Congratulate yourself! These small steps add up with time and consistency.

See your own beauty. You don't suddenly become beautiful after you lose another 50 pounds or from a new hairstyle or new clothes. Beauty comes from inside. It's not your shell, it's who you are.

Love thyself. Nothing worthwhile comes from a place of entrenched self-hatred. Maybe some old fashioned self-loathing got your attention to begin with, okay. But it's not a sustainable source of motivation and self-loathing is inherently at odds with behaving in a loving way towards your body.

Losing weight may change your collection of life experiences, but it doesn't change your core. By loving yourself, you affirm that your health and well-being is worth the effort and you deserve the best you can give yourself.

Taking care of yourself is selfish—in a good way! We so often ignore our own needs to care for others, forgetting that caring for the self must come first if you want to have any energy to devote to others.

Take time to celebrate your successes. You have many successes, every day! But we minimize, downplay, discount and ignore our successes so often, leaving us feeling inadequate and depressed.

Success is the most powerful weight loss drug imaginable, so start taking it daily.

Don't wait for the "Divine Bolt of Motivation" to strike. Sorry, but it's not happening. Hard things get started because we want to get them over and done with, or due consequences of not doing them, not because the Motivation Fairy visits in the night. Motivation does not proceed success; it follows it. Do something, anything—Just do! Then enjoy the feeling of progress, which does breed motivation.

You get what you focus on. If you want to be slender and healthy, don't focus on all the junk food you'd like to eat, or even how much you dislike being fat. You attract what you project; so project good stuff! Visualize success and every single day, acknowledge the gifts in your life with gratitude.

Changing your focus will change your life. Are you ready?!

CHAPTER 6

5 More Easy Steps to Lose the Tonnage

I was thinking the other day about the actual process I've gone through to lose the weight. (And if the PopTart queen can lose it, you can, too!)

People struggle needlessly. If you put out effort in the right ways, you can avoid the struggles and reap the rewards more easily. Let's skip the danger zones and zero right in on the rewards, shall we?

So in the hopes of helping you get started, here are five simple steps that got me moving.

Believing it was possible. THIS had to come before anything else. If you don't think it's possible, there's no drive to try, right? Now, I got there by starting to read success stories. I read tons of them. But more than that, it was the before and after pictures, with people as big or bigger than me. After about 5,002 pictures, something clicked in that brain of mine. "Hey! Just maybe I could do this, too!"

Preparation. This is not a code word for "avoidance" like it's so often used. Read up! Get informed! And figure out what you need. In other words, get the book Sparky!

This prep phase can last anywhere from a few days to a week or two. You're not trying to split the atom, man. But do know what you're doing.

Now: Do something! This is where, for me at least, it was critical that I didn't judge those early efforts at all. While I was still prepping, I simply started cutting down on sugar. Tapering off my Dr. Pepper habit. I went from buying 12-packs to buying a 2-liter to buying a 1-liter, and drinking it less all the time.

Was I "low-carbing?" Heck no! Was I making important changes and improving my odds for success? You bet your butt! The thing was, I was making relatively painless but VERY important changes that would start leading me down the right path. It was a start.

Be positive! This is a MAJOR and vastly underrated component of success. Why aren't people more positive? Maybe it's fear of disappointment or feeling stupid. But whatever the reason, forget that. Instead, EXPECT to succeed. Be positive. Hang out with supportive, positive people. Visualize yourself healthier. Really FEEL every accomplishment and relish it. Celebrate every accomplishment, even if silently.

If you sit around saying, "I can't pass up cookies, I can't control myself, blah, blah, blah, freakin' blah," well, you know what? You are programming your mind for failure.

However, if you say, "Wow, I'm doing great! I've improved this and this and that, and I feel great, and I look better every day and I'm amazing!"...Well that, my friends, has a much different effect.

Say what you want about all this positive thinking advice, but based on what I've observed, this component alone can make or break your success potential.

Build on successes and keep going. See, you're not even starting from scratch here! You already have success to build upon, from your getting prepared work, and you know it's success and feel good about it, since you've been staying positive and hanging out with positive people.

And when you've made a poor choice for some reason? Well, so what? That means NOTHING in the face of your obvious progress. It means you can use that situation to learn and adjust to help going forward.

It's effort, but it shouldn't be struggle. Do you see the difference? Effort is work, struggle is pain. Expect to work, and accept the work. But do not accept the pain. The pain is not necessary and it gets in the way.

But really, it's not even bad work. After you get started, it feels so great and there are SO MANY positive payouts, it's hard to think of it as anything but pure joy.

So start on your joy path already!

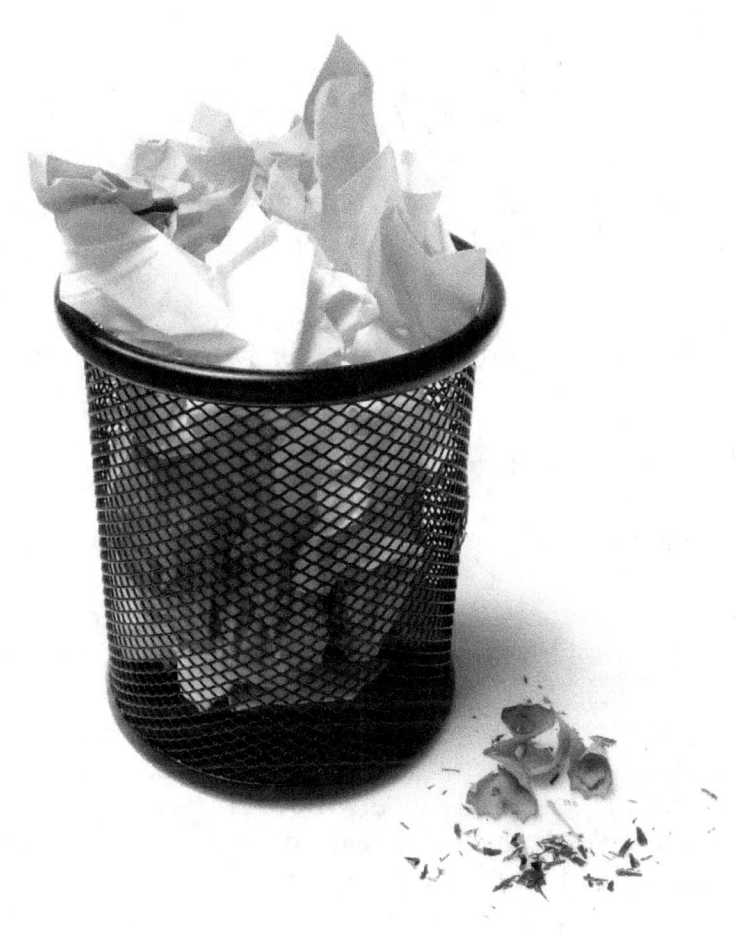

For the Back-Again Crowd

CHAPTER 7

What's Stopping You?

I heard a story about someone who got off track for a good while, and how she found her way back. The story itself doesn't matter too much, because so many of us already know it: she wasn't doing her plan, but couldn't say exactly why. There was always this little thing or that little thing, whatever it was, getting in the way. So she'd surely do it "soon." Except soon didn't seem to ever show up.

Sound familiar?

Personally, I suspect this is phase two of the "Diet Detour" that trips up even long-term, dedicated and smart dieters. Phase one is the creep, perhaps beget by bargaining ("a little won't hurt"), becoming gradually more frequent until you're not really on your plan much at all anymore. Maybe you still believe. You may still have the faith, sisters and brothers. But you're not practicing.

So you feel guilty. You chastise yourself and maybe get disgusted. And feeling as crummy and out-of-control as you do, you look to soothe that burn with a little more junk food comfort eating, followed by promises you'll restart "soon." You even mean it. But somehow, that soon never arrives.

Well, why not do something now, then? Now is super soon, after all. You want to get back on that wagon?

Here are some easy-to-follow tips for folks wanting to get back on track. Mix and match. Pick whatever appeals to you and just get yourself restarted already, for goodness sakes! You've got a life to live, y'kno.

Start improving your habits, whatever shape they may be in, RIGHT THIS MINUTE. You don't have to exercise three hours a day for it to count as an improvement. Fifteen minutes of activity is an improvement over none, and far more manageable than hours at a time. Maybe your eating isn't clean, but you can start avoiding the worst of the worst, right? Even if you're not fully back in the swing, you can get the ingredients for some of your on-plan favorites and add them to the menu rotation, right? Just freakin' start, man.

Stop asking yourself what's "wrong" with you. There's no inherent character flaw causing detours. Stress, illness, injury, business, family, whatever all distract us sometimes. You know? Any combination thereof. There are myriads of reasons people detour. The guilt-tripping just makes it harder to keep your attitude positive. By now, you know that's crucial, right? 'Cause it is, man!

Take care of your other needs (both physical and emotional). I harp on this, because I think self-care is usually the first item on the schedule to get cut and the last to be restored. Commitments to others always take precedence. What a waste: when we care for our own needs, we are SO much better equipped to help others, it's just a no-brainer. Love thyself first.

Set the stage for success. What helped you before? Did you cook ahead? Have some favorite snacks on hand? Haul around your favorite water jug everywhere? Happily while away the hours perusing new recipes? You don't have to be fully in the zone to start doing some of the stuff that helped you stay on track when you were on track.

Start knocking down obstacles. Look at what situations create the most problems for you, and start there. If friends have desserts at get-togethers, start bringing your own, plan-friendly dessert. (Others may appreciate this as well.) If you can't pass your spouse's snacks, buy a flavor or type you don't like. If you tend to overeat when you're tired or stressed, start addressing the tired and stressed issues, and the eating part falls into line.

Please stop calling the sugar-encrusted junk food "treats." I know this is how we've referred to them for years. I still do it sometimes, too. But when what you're really treating yourself is less health, is "treat" really how you want to describe it? Would it sound as appealing if we called them "fat pills" instead of "delicious donut hole treats?" Mentally connect what you're eating with what it creates. Not feeling your best is NOT a treat!

Remember: It wasn't that hard when you were in the zone. Remind yourself. I know of almost no one who has done this for any length of time who found it remotely as difficult as anticipated beforehand. With the huge variety of options and recipes, there is no excuse to be bored or unsatisfied with your food. Developing workable habits takes some time and effort initially, but soon become second nature.

Reread your plan. There will be bits and pieces you've forgotten, and just reviewing the material helps build motivation and resolve.

Participate in a community (like Low Carb Zen on Facebook). Even if you're not currently eating well, interacting with others who are will help inspire you. Seeing what they are talking about will also help remind you of the tricks of the trade, and why you decided to do it in the first place.

Think about the people who love and count on you. While people always say "you have to lose weight for yourself," considering loved ones can be some of the most powerful motivation available. Staying healthy and strong allows you to look forward to a longer, brighter future together. Setting a good example for your kids may significantly alter their lifestyles and health for the rest of their lives. It really is the absolute best gift you can give loved ones, taking good care of yourself.

Look for progress and celebrate it. Perfection isn't necessary (and its quest often becomes nothing more than a fancy method of procrastination). Any progress contributes positively to the sum total. There is NO improvement that's too small to build upon. It all counts.

Don't stop. If I had to sum up the secret to any and all dieting success in two words, those are the two! Don't stop. The only real failure is to give up on improving your health and your life. You're coherent enough to read these words? Then you've still got some kick left. Don't stop. Don't stop. Don't stop.

Focus on what you've got. A life of denial and restriction gets old fast. A life of enthusiasm and anticipation inspires and energizes. While this obviously applies to your menu, if you actually focus your attention on what you like about the rest of your life, it will help you be a happier person as well as a happier dieter. Happy people do better.

For many, detours ARE just another part of the journey. So treat it that way. Be kind to yourself and build yourself up. Give yourself permission to address your own needs, and remember that eating well is one of those needs that pays off so many ways.

Encourage yourself along the same way you would a beloved friend, and you can't go too far astray.

And welcome home.

CHAPTER 8

Back on Track?

You've fallen and you're not sure if you want to get up, huh?

Listen. Everyone who has struggled with weight has had those days. Maybe you have been eating junk for a day or three...or thirty, whatever. You're tired of thinking about everything you put in your mouth, and ask yourself if maybe life wasn't so bad when your biggest food worry was not running out of Oreos. This has been hard, and you loved your sugar...

Well, stop that right now! And please, don't tell me you can't because that's a load of bull hockey. As long as you are saying you can't, I believe you. When you start saying you can, it's possible. Until then, it's not. So don't waste any more time, and come back when you're ready to move on.

Still here? Okay, Sparky. I can work with that. Let's go!

What kills people in their attempts to lose weight is NOT the occasional off-plan eating, although it often starts there. One isolated incident of poor eating choices means NOTHING beyond whatever meaning you give it. The choices you make day in and day out is what will bear the fruit.

What gets people is the interpretation they give their off-plan incidents.

But if you continue to give it the same meaning that most of us have, especially every OTHER time we'd tried to lose weight and failed...well, where are you headed? And by that I mean this circular, self-defeating thinking spiral-as in, "What's wrong with me? I can't believe I blew it," and on and on and on. It's not a personality defect that derails anybody. It's that darned thinking!

Truth is, you ain't blown diddley! If you were discussing a "diet," where you have a specific set of rules and broke the rules, hence losing the contest, okay, whatever. You expect total perfection, you guarantee yourself failure eventually.

But you're not talking about a diet. You're talking about your life, for goodness sakes! You are changing your eating habits for L-I-F-E, life. Which means there will be times when you make a few less advisable choices. So what? Just keep the on-track choices far outnumbering the off-track ones.

But instead, if you stop and berate yourself over perceived flaws, you talk yourself right out of doing the work you need to do. You decide it's just beyond you, throw up your hands and give up. That's no good!

I actually find it encouraging when someone reaches the point they normally would have given up before. That's not as weird as it seems.

If you are considering giving up, it points to one, very important fact: You're at a crossroads. This is probably a place where you have given up in the past, what stopped you before. Right?

Which means you now have the OPPORTUNITY to decide where this goes from here. You can lick that demon, man! This is the place for the Phoenix to rise. Let your old, unsuccessful "dieting" identity die off, to be replaced by your new way of life. That is why THIS time can work, will work, when other times did not work. You take a different path at the crossroad. That is a powerful position to be in, man!

Banish the word "can't" from your weight loss vocabulary. Replace it with "choice." Even if you don't believe this 100%, your subconscious will hear you telling yourself it is all a choice and the process will begin.

You can't change your pants size until you change what goes on in your head. And don't fool yourself for a minute: it IS a process, not an event. You are learning new habits and breaking old ones. Change is challenging!

But the truth is, once we let go of some of the problematic attitudes that helped keep us overweight, the other stuff starts to magically fall into place. It's kind of like sex that way: it all begins and ends in your head. The other stuff is just (primal, keto, low-carb) dressing, man.

Ask yourself: what led me off-track? When did I first start noticing I was sliding into old habits? Were there warning signs? How did I feel? If you can use this insight to develop your own early-warning system and make the straying time an asset, not a problem.

I know it's extra tough when you're under a lot of stress, but get focused and what you'll find is that once you get over the hump of some temporary discomfort that comes from changing long-ingrained habits...well, you'll actually greatly RELIEVE your stress by making good eating choices. You will feel better and I can promise you this: feeding your body healthy food will help you deal with stress way more effectively than sugar ever did! Taking care of yourself helps you be in a position to take care of everything and everyone else, too.

Having a rough time, right now? Here's what to do.

Remind yourself of successes. It seems counter-intuitive maybe, but that is EXACTLY where you need to focus when you're feeling upset with yourself. 'Cause bad feelings lead to poor choices. Success, on the other hand, leads to more success.

Say nice stuff to yourself! People think they will start to feel better about themselves once they lose weight. That's backwards. You start to lose weight once you start to feel better about yourself. I'm 100% serious about this one. It works.

Remind yourself why you're doing it all, anyway. Maybe you've got a family and you want to be around for them. More than you know, your choices will impact their choices and even health over time. And especially if you have kids who need to lose weight: they don't need for you to be perfect. But they need for you to hang in there with them and help them see what's possible by leading the way.

Getting back on the wagon IMMEDIATELY. Don't make the arbitrary and meaningless distinctions that "today is shot" or the weekend or week or month or whatever is somehow ruined. Your backside doesn't check the calendar. Your life is made of up individual moments. Address each one as it comes up and the future takes form all by itself.

Have many backup plans and coping skills ready to spring into action. Forget willpower, which is useless anyway. It comes and goes...like the tide. Bah. My money is on planning every time!

Journaling is a big help for many. You have lots of processing going on as you change your body and your life. So process it. You are starting to eat like a thinner person, so start THINKING like a thinner person, too. Emotions are a big part of this puzzle.

Think positive, self-supportive thoughts. Take the Pollyanna challenge: stop yourself every time you hear a negative self-assessment and replace it with a positive spin instead. Support yourself by hanging with positive people. You will attract what you focus on. Make sure that's it is not snack cakes you're focusing on, dude!

I'm of the opinion that it doesn't matter how many slips you have. This isn't a race, it's your life.

The only thing that matters is that you keep coming back, consistent and persistent. If you make 1000 mistakes, then come back 1001 times.

I imagine there is not a single person undertaking a major change who hasn't felt distraught enough to consider giving up at some point along the way. But you CAN break through it. You just have to ride it out and replace any pain and struggle with positive thoughts and emotions.

Healthy eating is an amazing tool, and it has indeed changed my life. But I am without question in this realization: If I hadn't adjusted my attitude along with my eating, I'd have failed utterly.

When you're feeling off-kilter and in danger, read some uplifting material or pull out some of your motivational books or write of list of all the ways you're a great person or call a friend or take a walk or go out and just breathe in the scents of trees and flowers. Whatever you do, lift your mood. Then visualize yourself successful, focus on your successes, and think about successes.

Realize wherever you're at now is okay. Understand, you may be crashing and burning because this is what NEEDS to happen. Your old ways hadn't gotten you to where you want to be, right? Sometimes, crisis or pain arrives to shake things up. Maybe, you needed more understanding, to "kill off" your old behavior style as you outgrow it.

Take it as a lesson you evidently needed before you're able to move past. Maybe this crossroads cropped up exactly because you are doing the work you need to do.

And yes, sometimes it's challenging. But maybe you are facing this particular challenge precisely because mastering it is exactly what's required for you to take this whole enterprise to the next level.

I think it's that one.

The point is, we all go down sometimes. When you go down, you can either stay down, or you can come back up with a new understanding, better prepared than ever. You can be a dead ducky or the Phoenix, rising more powerful than ever before.

Which do you pick?

(Unnecessary Hint: I'm rooting for the Phoenix!)

CHAPTER 9

Dieting with a History of Eating Disorders

Many have struggled with unwanted pounds (and the physical and emotional ramifications of those pounds), in some cases for decades. Like me. Probably most of us in that position have tried numerous ill-advised and, in some cases, outright dangerous schemes to ditch the weight.

I did. You don't qualify as "morbidly obese" for 35 years of your life without trying a few traditional and not-so-traditional "solutions," after all. Some led me to lose a few pounds in the short term, but none of them allowed me to keep off what I'd lost. As soon as I quit the excessive behavior, the pounds came back in force.

Therefore, I understand the desperation that brings people to this place, very well. I understand intimately what it means to live life as a fat chick. I know it's no fun.

So it's not a surprise to me that folks come to weight loss support communities with similar history and baggage. In some cases, the more extreme weight loss efforts would qualify for a clinical diagnosis of an Eating Disorder (ED).

Eating behavior is on a continuum, and most people don't make it here without having spent at least some time in an unhealthy range of that continuum. Maybe you're not there yet, but you could be moving in that direction. Either way, it's no way to live.

But I'm offering you a way out, if you're prepared to take it. You can continue the same maladaptive behavior you've tried in the past, just substituting extreme low-carb / Paleo / whatever as your culinary punishment of choice...and expect the same kind of results. Or you could get a handle on your eating and perspective, to find a healthy, sustainable way to manage your health and weight for the rest of your life.

Here's how:

If you need help managing your emotional state and perceptions surrounding eating and weight, GET it. If your picture of yourself is "fat" inside your head, no amount of weight dropped can change that. Body image is multifaceted, almost all of it unrelated to what the rest of the world sees. And I can promise you that if those emotional issues are not resolved, there is NO magic number on the scale that will erase the pain. This has to come first.

Discontinue extreme/compulsive behaviors with eating and food immediately. (And if you can't manage this on your own, get help before you even attempt to undertake any eating plan.) This includes purging, binging, frenzied exercise, compulsive fasting, etc. You know what I'm talking about if this is an issue for you.

Please stop calling yourself "fat, disgusting, lazy, stupid," etc. ad infinitum. That's not true and it just makes me really, really sad. It also makes it much harder for you to take good care of yourself. If self-denigration worked for weight loss, fat people would be virtually nonexistent.

After you get a single, starting baseline, pack the scale and tape measure away. For most with a history of ED-related issues, these are powerful triggers that can spiral them into depression and self-disgust. Religiously stay away from anything that you know triggers excessive behavior. Don't allow yourself to pull these out again except at predefined intervals, and then only if you decide it's safe for you. (Once a month, for example, would be reasonable – NOT daily)! Keep them at a friend's house. Put them in a storage locker. Throw them out. I don't care what you do with these things, just don't let them run your life. If it makes you feel bad or triggers you, avoid it.

Pick a reputable, established healthy eating plan, and follow it to the letter. Don't "sort of, mostly" follow it. Don't eat less than the plan outlines to lose weight faster (which doesn't work, by the way), or don't eat more sometimes and later nothing to cancel out that "weakness." (And if all you care about is losing weight and not what the process does to your body, this is still the best way to do it; eating erratically can actually stop losses as your body tries to compensate and eventually, you can damage your metabolism to the point that it becomes all but impossible to lose weight, ever.)

Focus ONLY on progress. The only real failure is to give up, so by definition, if you're doing your best to take care of yourself, you ARE successful. Progress comes in many forms, by the way. Scales, measurements and clothing sizes are one way to measure. Energy level and overall health are other ways. This will be a challenge, but well worth it. In fact, the most reliable indicator of long-term success I see consistently is a positive attitude. Positive thinking does work!

Monitor your emotional state, and get additional professional support as needed. While online or real life communities can provide you with peer support for your eating plan, this is not the same as spending time with a therapist who understands treating EDs and can help you cope with that and other challenging areas of your life.

Now, I happen to believe low carb, Keto or Paleo any one can make a solid, long-term choice for people who have ED-related issues, provided they have reached a place where they are able to follow an established plan without compulsive behaviors.

This way of eating, faithfully followed, get cravings under control, manages hunger, and leaves adherents with lots of energy and overall improved health. But if you use low carb or it's kin as just another version of the crash-diet-of-the-week and persist in extreme behaviors that wreak havoc with your system, you put yourself right back where you were before, still struggling, still feeling awful, and still slowly (or quickly) killing yourself. Please don't associate that with these diet plans.

I realize everyone has to make their own choices and your decisions are always your own, whether I agree or not. But Eating Disorders are something I take very seriously; the sad truth is that people die from eating disorders! I care about the folks that look to the work I do for support.

So if you have active ED concerns, please don't just tell yourself you can just "use them" for a little while to lose the weight or that the behavior doesn't count if you hide it. Your issues will not become magically resolved when the scale hits your happy zone. The issues aren't stored in the fat cells, okay? Get the professional support you need to live a healthy life.

You do have a choice. I hope you choose to care enough about yourself and your loved ones to do whatever work necessary to live free from the demons and obsessions of Eating Disorders. It can be done and it's very, very worth it.

I'm rooting for you!

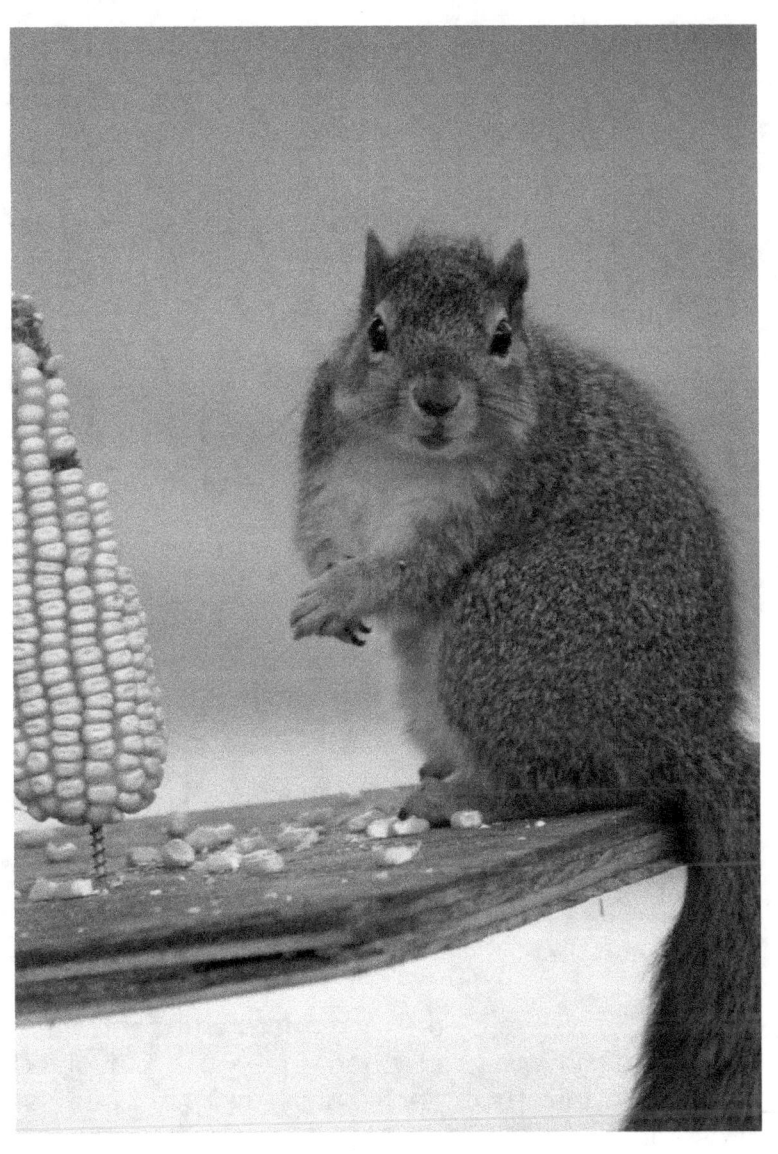

Off-Plan Eating

CHAPTER 10

Planning on Eating Illegal

There is a place in your plan for off-plan eating, provided you've planned it! Maybe you won't agree, but hear me out and maybe you will.

First of all, I have one completely incontrovertible rule for all off-plan eating: It must be planned. That sounds ironic, doesn't it? Off-plan planning. I made a funny.

No matter what you put in your mouth, I want you to think about it beforehand. I want you to make thought-out, informed decisions about everything you eat. Why? You have a better chance of succeeding—that's why!

When you eat off-plan because of a spur-of-the-moment circumstance—the smell of food in a mall, or spying one of your old favorites on the potluck table, for example—then it's already turning into an impulsive act.

Impulsive acts are by their very nature uncontrolled. They don't involve reflection. They don't involved making an informed decision by weighing out the pros and cons. They just kind of "happen" and tend to make folks feel out-of-control. Like you're submitting, right? Giving up? Giving in?

On the other hand, let's say you have a particular occasion coming up. It's your anniversary, a kid's birthday. Whatever. There is a situation where you would like to drink a glass of wine or eat a few bites of cake or whatnot. (Wine is fine, but no whine, please! I'm allergic to whine.)

So you decide, you're going to eat off-plan for this occasion, in a way and amount that doesn't significantly disrupt your long-term health goals.

It's vital you don't feel deprived or sorry for yourself. That's setting yourself up for a fall. It's vital you feel like you can live with your plan and integrate it into your lifestyle. Sometimes, this may mean you make a decision to eat a limited amount of something that would divert you from your goals with regular consumption.

In a situation where you've made a decision about eating illegally, you know what's coming. You've thought it out, considered the consequences, and have decided it fits into your acceptable risk zone. You have decided beforehand what you're going to eat and how much. You've made the plans you need to do this successfully. You adjust your intake to compensate earlier in the day. You drink extra water, and get a little exercise in. You plan to stay off the scale for the next few days, since you anticipate the potential of an ascending scale dial common after off-plan eating because of water retention.

"Be-Informed" Sidebar: People don't physically gain 5 pounds of fat after an illegal eating incident. But you can gain five pounds of water immediately. After you eat low-carb for a while for example, your body responds differently to digesting carbs, including some serious water retention. So don't freak out. Watching people freak out makes me very, very tired.

But even more important than the prep factor— by only eating off-plan when you've decided to beforehand, you are giving yourself the message that YOU are in control. This isn't about feeling as if you couldn't resist. (Cookie Godfather visit?) This isn't because you have inadequate willpower. (Willpower is a silly concept, anyway. How about Planning Power instead?)

Unplanned illegal eating gives you the exact wrong message: You can't do it. It doesn't stimulate feelings of mastery and self-control, that's for sure! What kind of things do you tell yourself then? You're weak? You can't make it? You'll never reach your goals?

No, no, no! Your self-definition is what drives your reality. You will ultimately act in accordance with how you self-define.

The other thing about unplanned illegal eating: It's uncontrolled. You're much more likely to decide to chuck in the whole day, week, whatever if you are making decisions without thinking them through.

If you've told yourself beforehand, "Okay, I will have ½ of a Dessert-Thing and a couple tablespoons of Other-Thing," that's probably what you'll actually have. That's do-able and you remain in control.

Tips on Safe Illegal Eating

Make planned choices, legal or illegal. Consider pros, cons, and especially consequences.

Feel your own power in the process. Whether you're eating legally or illegally, YOU are the driving force. It's always better and more empowering to take responsibility than to pretend you're a victim of circumstance.

Control your choices. If you are gonna eat illegal, then decide beforehand how much and of what. That way, you're already outlined the scope of the incident. Don't consider anything else as an option.

If you do end up "losing it" with an illegal eating incident, take note! This does NOT need to be a huge problem. If you learn from the situation, if you use this information in making future choices, it can turn into a huge boon for your long-term success instead of a stumbling block. The more you know about yourself, the better prepped you are to be successful.

Compensate other ways to help yourself continue to feel in control. If you're gonna carb it up this weekend, eat fewer carbs a few days before. Don't go insane here, but maybe eat induction-style for a couple of days. Drink extra water. Be prepared and be smart.

Maybe the most important tip of all: Eat illegally infrequently. The choices you make most often are the ones that come home to roost. It is, as it always has been, 100% up to you.

And if you don't feel like you can eat a few bites and move on? Don't. You'll feel better in the morning. No matter what happens, keep your focus, stay real with yourself, and keep your brain engaged, and you'll be fine.

All this having been said? **I'm mostly going to suggest you avoid off-plan eating.** There are so many on-plan choices, so many ways you can remain on track and not feel deprived, I find very little to be gained from straying.

People say, "Life is short. Enjoy it!" I say, "Life is shorter and a lot less pleasant if I don't take care of myself. I want to enjoy it!"

Be careful (and mindful) out there!

CHAPTER 11

Cheating and Other Aberrations

I sometimes hear people talk about cheating...how they screwed everything up, blew up, lost it, etc. etc.

And it bugs the heck out of me! Ok, so you eat one thing that's high carb (or whatever tune your drummer plays), and you're done? Your life is over?

You've just messed up everything completely and utterly?

"Oh well, let's throw up my hands and give up now, since I've discovered I wasn't 100% perfect like I thought I was? That being human thing is for losers. I'm better than that..."

Get over yourself already! Who died and elected you perfect? Now, I understand that mindset. I do. Oh lord, how I understand it...

How do you think I got fat in the first place? It was "too hard," it "wasn't worth it," and "I screwed everything all up and may as well forget it anywho." Yeah. That's exactly what happened. And you know what? That mindset will make you fat, too!

Well Holy Moly. Talk about having difficulties with delayed gratification...There is basically only one way to blow it as far as I'm concerned...stop! That's it.

If you stop working on your issues and you stop trying to improve, then yes, you've blown it. But since you can restart again any time, then you effectively have until you die to do it. You ain't dead yet, baby! So stop acting like it.

I dunno. I just think if you eat a plate of French fries, then, okay. You ate some French Fries. Digest and move on already. Is there some reason this must become a major emotional challenge?

Here's what you can do constructively. Think about how it makes you feel physically and emotionally. Decide if it's a way you like to feel. Think about whether or not it's in line with what your long term goals. And if it's not, then you'll be armed with that knowledge next time you face down a plate of fries, right?

But don't bother with the wailing and the gnashing of teeth, all Biblical style. Just stay away from the fries, Sparky.

I don't mean to be insensitive. Well, OK. I'm not worrying about sensitivity too much. But that's not the point. I guess the thing is, I can just see it all so clearly now, this time around.

Look at the words we use, even. "Cheat." Cheating implies breaking the rules, doing something undetected, in secret. Who or what exactly, are we cheating? Dr. Atkins? Your beef jerky will realize you're seeing other snacks?

Here's why I think it's called cheating: we're trying to sneak food past our brains, so our butt won't notice and react with weight gain. You think if you don't say it very loud, your behind won't hear what you ate.

Ever heard somebody talk who "got away" with a cheat? It's almost like a kid who snuck past the principal to ditch school—pretending like your backside won't know what your mouth is packing away if you whisper is ridiculous.

The whole thing becomes some kind of bizarre mind game. And the mentality gets to me sometimes. "Oh my God. I've cheated and I'm so bad and I am so lost and clueless and I have no control over myself and whatever shall I do?!"

And it may not surprise you that I have an answer. I'm sorry, but it's time to grow up. You aren't being force fed. (And this advice applies to myself, too, by the way. I understand it because I've been guilty of it!)

What will it take for people to realize that what to have for dinner is not a MORAL decision? Do you call your Religious Counsel to discuss appetizers? I didn't think so, and if you do, your issues are beyond the scope of my expertise, anywho. Get thee to a psychiatric office, posthaste.

Otherwise, realize that you are making choices. And some of those choices can lead down a road you don't want to travel.

Yes, some folks have medical issues. But me? I got fat because I ate too darned much. I have thyroid issues and family history that predisposes me to fatness, but I'm the chick that munched up those PopTarts, baby. Can't blame that on my metabolism or society.

Does that make me a bad person? Heck no! It makes me somebody who likes chocolate, dang it. But I like being healthy more than I like chocolate, so I'm on track. And if I pop a half a donut here or there? I'm not fooling anybody. My butt is still gonna know about it.

I'm not a bad person, though. I'm just a person who needs to keep track of what I eat if I want to get skinnier.

And the same goes for you.

CHAPTER 12

Cheating: Road to Freedom or Diet Plan Ruin?

Cheat days? Reward Meals? Time off-plan? Are these strategies a part of successful plan? Some think so; others don't. Before you make up your mind, consider the bigger picture.

Reward Meals

Newbies sometimes get confused about reward meals. Specifically, someone getting their info via word of mouth may hear about a "Reward Meal" and consider it part of what low carbing is about....there are even plans cropping up nowadays claiming "carb refeeds" are an essential part of success: an opportunity to eat whatever one wants once a day or week or whatever and still lose weight! Sounds great, right?

Personally, I think that's a load of bull hockey. Why? Most times I've heard reward meals discussed, the notion of restraint is conspicuously missing. It seems more of a "I've been good on my diet so I've earned a break" type function for many.

Cheat Days

Cheat days are—what else?—a day off the diet, where said participant ingests whatever they want.

Reward meals time three: an entire day (or more) of eating without rules. The best of both worlds? Literally having your (diet) cake and eating the traditional cake, too?

Some folks say that planning to have a vacation from their eating plan makes it easier for them to follow it the rest of the time. Others say it's an invitation for disaster. Which is it, for you?

What Are You Looking For?

Some frequently heard arguments in favor of the Cheat/Reward:

It helps me say "No" the rest of the time.
I'm doing well sticking to my plan, so I've earned it.
I just can't give up [insert-beloved-food-item-here], so this allows me to control it.
I want to be able to eat like everybody else.
I can always lose any weight I've put on by getting stricter on my plan.
Since this is a lifestyle and not a diet, there will be times I eat off-plan.
It hasn't kept me from losing.

Arguments against the Cheat:

It undoes progress you've made during the time you've remained faithful to your plan.
It can knock you out of Ketosis and eliminate some of the mad benefits: reduced appetite, increased energy and lack of cravings.

It reinforces the dieting mindset: your normal menu remains a form of deprivation, whereas unhealthy foods are defined as "treats" that are to be longed for.

Many people feel crummy physically after eating significantly more carbs than they are accustomed to consuming.

Sugar consumption can lead to addictive behavior and binges for many.

Off-plan eating can stimulate cravings and increased hunger for many.

A "little here and a little there" quickly adds up, until you find you're eating off-plan more and more. Carb creep, hello!

The Detox Link

I worked in a county detox for a few years. It was eye-opening, let me tell ya! I met people addicted to anything and everything you can imagine. I saw people who drank hair spray (for the alcohol content), or huffed spray paint until they couldn't string a coherent sentence together. I've even seen someone chug an entire bottle of Pepto Bismal and rinse out a nasal spray bottle with water to try and get another shot out of it.

In other words, I've seen addiction up close.

You notice something common to addicts watching them come and go (and very often, come back again): they bargain. A lot. They change the definitions of acceptable behavior to support the addiction, and create a set of rules in how they will partake as a means of trying to maintain an illusion of control.

Bargaining I heard on a daily basis at detox:

It's only beer so it doesn't count. You can't be an alcoholic if you only drink beer.
I don't do drugs. I just drink. (What do people think alcohol is besides a drug? Duh.)
I only use on weekends/when I'm stressed out/when I really need to/when somebody else does/etc. ad infinitum
I could cut back if I wanted to, so it's okay / I've already cut back, so it's okay.
I'm not as bad as some people I know. Other people can control it–so I can, too.
Since I'm going to treatment, [insert negative consequence of using] won't happen.

Seeing the dots yet?

Now, I'm not telling you that if you choose to go off-plan, you're an addict. What I am suggesting is that you ask the question. It's a worthy question.

If the answer is no, you have lost nothing by asking. If the answer is yes, you may have saved yourself much grief.

Just a little something to think about.

CHAPTER 13

The Brownies are Not in Charge!

"I caved. I ate that brownie. I couldn't resist."

These are not my confessions. This is what I hear people say when they're trying to lose weight. Be it brownies or fries or whatever. But one thing does far more damage than the eating: the attitude!

EVERY time you talk about "caving in, giving in, giving up, losing the battle, being unable to resist temptation," you are doing one thing you really, really don't want to do: programming the message into your brain that you are unable to lose weight.

You're surrendering your fate to a damned brownie!

Now, I don't actually give a flying rodent's backside whether you eat that brownie or not. It's not the one brownie, or 2 or even 5, although you'll probably feel crummy if you hit the 5...but it's not about whether or not you eat the brownie(s).

It's about CONTROL, responsibility, and your ability to stand up to brownies.

Aside: if you do eat that brownie, but you declare it a CHOICE, then you haven't given up your fate to an inanimate (although perhaps tasty) hunk of flour and sugar, you know? Who is in charge here, you or the Keebler elves? Who really has your best interests at heart?

See, the thing is, there is fallout for feeling like you just "can't" resist, too. Yeah, you get to eat what you want. But you also are telling yourself time and again you're weak, you're lazy, you disgusting and unworthy, you've got no willpower or whatever.

You keep telling yourself this garbage, and it's just a short trip to believing it, followed by to living it! 'Cause why even bother trying if you're doomed to failure anyway? You may be miserable and fat, but you'll have a mouthful of chocolate on the way down?

And it's not just eating the self-loathing impacts. Who is going to be revved up for exercise, for self care efforts? The person who sees themselves as disgusting, gross, needing redemption and is looking at exercise as a punishment, or the person who feels in control, happy, and just wants to be healthier? Pain versus pleasure, my money's on the pleasure every time.

That self-loathing spiral is what turns a couple of off-plan eating incidents into a 2 month weight-gain extravaganza. It's WAY in your best interests to make this simple shift of taking responsibility.

Is change hard? Sure. To a point. (It's usually much less hard than we expect.) But it's a choice. Initially, any new behavior is always going to be somewhat uncomfortable. Personally, I think it's worth suffering some temporary discomfort while developing new habits.

But no matter what you decide, about your brownie or what's an acceptable size for your own butt long-term, please don't whimper about giving in to irresistible forces, okay? While it could appear that way to the casual observer, truth is there isn't a tractor beam from your mouth to the brownie plate.

Give yourself the gift of not abandoning your power to a hunk of food, for goodness sakes. Take responsibility on every level by acknowledging your DECISIONS are running the show, not the irresistible forces of brownie magic.

Program the message instead that you ARE in control, you decide what you eat, and you decide what efforts you're making for your health and your future.

Stay in the driver's seat and you can make it to your destination my friends. It's worth the trouble!

CHAPTER 14

Confessions of a Carb Addict

When I first heard of low carb, it only took one sentence for me to know I had zero interest: "no bread, no pasta, no sugar."

I responded, "No way!"

These people were obviously insane if they thought there was a chance in Hades I was going to give all that up. I simply could not imagine my life without this type of food. I lived for bread. I actually made a point of buying food with sugar in it: the more, the better. I'd start getting antsy if we only had one box of snack cakes in the house, and God help us if we actually ran out.

I didn't know it at the time, but yes, I was an addict.

But it gets worse.

You know why I did start taking low carb seriously? I was told I could expect to develop diabetes any minute. It ran in both sides of my family and at my weight, looked inevitable. So in the end, I ended up getting serious about low carb—and stopped eating sugar—because I was terrified of not being able to eat sugar anymore. Oh, the irony!

Somehow, I didn't put two and two together, figured I'd diet my way out of this fix and get on with my life. Just eat less junk later. Right?

Yeah. I'm sure you know where that's going.

Well, after I started experiencing some success, low carb started to click for me. One of the switches that went off in my head was the realization that "diet" is a dirty word, because it means temporary struggle directed toward temporary ends. I didn't want to go back. I still don't.

So forget the temporary ends! And the struggle inherent in the dieting concept is rooted in feelings of restriction and denial. But it needn't be, because this bit is utterly voluntary. My thinking changed and it made all the difference.

And I haven't gone back, but I will tell you in all honesty, I've taken a few steps back. I've lost some 125 pounds, and over the past few years, regained some of it. Not all by any means, but too much. Ouch. And I'll can tell you exactly how I reversed some of my own hard-won losses in a single word: bargaining!

"Just a little won't hurt. I need it because I'm tired/stressed/angry/whatever. If I only buy a single serving package, it's okay. It's still a lot better than I used to eat. If I don't do it every day, then it's not a problem. Everybody else is having some. I deserve a treat. If I put on a couple pounds, I know how to lose them. I've done it before."

The list goes on and on, my friend. Recognize any of 'em?

But not everything I did was a mistake. I never stopped. I never stopped considering myself a low carber, even when I knew my eating wasn't what it could be. I always considered any off-plan eating as temporary, even when the sloppy habits drug on for months and added on to my hips. And I saved myself a lot of pain that way.

But I am STILL on the journey. Friends say, "Dixie, you won't go back to your old weight. You worked too hard to lose it.""

I want to agree with them—I'd really like to—but I know better. It's not an impossibility. Just like people believe if they have lost the weight, they can lose it again...well, I believe if I have carried the weight, I can carry it again.

It doesn't happen overnight. It doesn't smack you in the face at the time. It's insidious and sneaky. It certainly was as the scale climbed up. I didn't ever expect ever get that fat...who does? But it can happen, because it did!

And I didn't expect to regain an ounce of what I lost. But I did. Instead of wasting time feeling sorry for myself however, I am determined to use my experiences to help myself—and, I hope, help you!

I can't answer the off-plan question for you, any more than I can tell you if you can stop at one drink in a bar.

I can give you the answer for me, though—remaining at a healthy weight for me is much more

REWARDING than eating junk that makes me gain weight and feel lousy. Making the effort to take care of myself is a lot more pleasant than the effort it would take to address one of the multitude of obesity-related health complications that were a part of my alternate future.

I won't tell you I'll never eat something off-plan again, because I'd be a liar. But I sure can tell you that I take the choice much more seriously than I used to, courtesy some backsliding reality checks borne from bargaining.

I guess it depends on your definition of freedom. I'm not willing to cheat myself out of the true path to freedom I've found in eating healthy.

May each of us find our own path to freedom, and relish the journey along the way.

CHAPTER 15

10 Reasons Your Diet Didn't Work (& Fixes)

I'm a Low Carb evangelist, no doubt about it. I love promoting low carb because I'd like to give others the same gift I've gotten. As a side effect of my ministry, I'm often told by folks that they've "tried that once, but it didn't work."

I've noticed a number of common mistakes or misunderstandings that very consistently cause problems. I talk about low carb because that's my thing, but the same is true of other dietary approaches. Learn the pitfalls and you can effectively avoid 'em.

Not having a plan. This is the number #1 mistake I see. So many people either a) simply stop eating carbs altogether (Errr...what about veggies, friend? It wasn't the broccoli that made your hips swell!); or b) take a friend's word for what the plan is all about. I don't care if your friend did great with their version. I mean, sure, I wish 'em well and all! But 99% of the time, the info from a friend is incomplete, flawed, and altered to fit the friend's personal inclinations. Go to the source.

Not buying the book. You can't be "doing Atkins" if you don't have the book! No pass go, no collecting $200. The people who pick a plan and buy the book for their plan do better across the board. To be honest, I've never seen someone who refused this step last more than a few weeks before abandoning their plan as "not working." Informed people do better. Do your homework!

Not giving it a chance. For most people, the first week is tough. Maybe very tough! The more carbs you had been consuming prior, the tougher it is. As your body goes through withdrawal, you will likely feel like death warmed over. Once you get through those withdrawals however, and transform yourself into a fat-burning machine, most people report feeling better than they have in years–with lots more energy, less appetite, and reduced physical complaints. Isn't that worth holding out the first few days of Induction/Keto/Paleo flu?

Ignoring the plan, selectively. Sure, I get it. I bent Atkins when I started, and it still worked for me, well enough that I eventually got more serious about compliance. But the more you bend it, the less likely your results will be consistent. Let's face it: if your very own, snowflake special, do-it-yourself eating plan was working so well, would you be here now?

Frankenfoods, man. Low carb specialty foods we often call "Frankenfoods." That should give you a clue of how I see them. Be informed and be aware. Junk food with "low carb" or "Paleo" slapped on the label is still junk food, and the food manufacturers are looking at their bottom line, not our health. The most dangerous from what I've seen are the sweets (as sugar alcohols can be very problematic) and carb bars, which are the number one source of mysterious stalls I've seen around weight loss communities. The shakes are not as troublesome for most, but it's always an individual question what foods cause problems for you personally. You have to experiment for yourself.

Not utilizing recipes. I know you may not be a cook. Lord knows I'm not! But if this is going to be your new way of life (and if you don't want to regain the weight, it'd better be), you need to know how to make satisfying food, on-plan style. The more natural the food, the better you'll do. Which means getting over any kitchen phobia. You don't have to be a great cook, but you have to be willing to try, at least a little. Adapting favorites and having lots of options is exactly what keeps you from feeling deprived.

Not reading the labels. Successful dieters are compulsive label readers. Sugar is the enemy, and even if the carb count works for you, if it has sugar, consider keeping it out of your mouth. There is no replacement for informed decisions.

Not tracking. I hate tracking, with a passion. So I also get this. Whooooo boy. But I also know my eyeball estimation of a serving is way different than what the food scale says, and my "what I ate today" ball-parking is way different from what I get when I actually keep score. If I'm struggling, I know this is where I need to go. Study after study bears out the truth, people who track lose more weight. It's sort of like doing a budget to track spending. It hurts a minute, but man, does it help long term.

Giving up too soon. Nutrition and the body's response to dietary changes is a highly individual process. A food that causes only 1% of dieters trouble can be an issue if you're part of that 1%. Test, rinse, repeat. Ask for help. Listen to your body. It gives you the clues via how you feel

Going it alone. Another success factor borne out by the research repeatedly is that dieters who utilize a support community are more successful.

I can vouch personally, had I not sought out and found community in the early stages of my own journey, I would not have been nearly as successful. It was the real world advice that took me to the next level.

You get the perspective and encouragement from the community. You get tips, tricks, ideas, and a friendly word on the day you most need it. You get people who understand and who aren't going to tell you to shut up about the diet already. It really does matter.

CHAPTER 16

How to Fail at Losing Weight

In the course of my own journey, I've gotten the opportunity to observe a lot of people. Some have been very successful, while others fizzle out in a matter of minutes, it seems. I notice some behaviors and traits frequently seem to precede impending doom for weight loss!

Here's a quick rundown of how to defeat yourself as you're trying to lose weight, in my not-so-humble opinion.

Sabotage Your Weight loss Efforts by...

...Telling yourself constantly what you can't have. I mean, c'mon. You CAN have whatever you want to. It's just some choices lead to what you're looking for, and some don't. If you make more "squishy" choices, then guess where you're heading?

...Feeling sorry for yourself! What the Heck? I see no reason to feel sorry for myself. I ate the dang brownies to begin with, so I can work 'em off. If your most pressing problem is munchies for some chocolate cake, count your blessings, brothers and sisters!

...Hanging around off-plan food. Spending lots of time preparing it, looking at it, sitting nearby while other people are eating it, wistfully sniffing if...well heck. Like the sober alcoholic that is always at the neighborhood bar, the sugar-addict that ogles chocolate cake is halfway in route to jumping off the wagon.

...Not having a plan! Get the book, for goodness sakes. You can't afford NOT to get the book. Pick a plan, get the book and get this party started. I don't care what worked for your co-worker's ex-mother-in-law or who gave you the list of what to eat. Just get the dang book already!

...Imparting a moral status to eating behavior. Food is not broken down into good and bad. While some food is good for you or not-so-good for you, morality is not embedded within the food itself. Food is neither enemy or friend. You are NOT good or bad person based on what you eat, okay? Please stop looking at it that way. It just makes me sad.

...Being helpless. If you're helpless in the face of cravings, or outside pressure, or lack of family support or whatever else your issue is, you're not going anywhere. (At least not anywhere you like.) If somebody is holding a gun to your head while they shove cookies in your mouth, okay. You can claim helpless. Otherwise, let's get real.

...Visualizing failure. Sitting around and constantly telling yourself you can't do this, or even just questioning your ability to succeed, is the best way to ensure you don't! If you focus on failing, that's what you're going to do. If you focus on success and visualize success, it becomes more real every minute.

...Asking yourself if you can give up your personal "magic food" for the rest of your life. Yeah, that's right. While I do emphasize this is a permanent change to lifestyle—and rightly so—you are NOT dealing with the rest of your life. When you look at all of anything in the context of the rest of your life, it's overwhelming. Ever think about how much you're going to have to work, the rest of your life? Or how much cleaning you'll have to do, the rest of your life? You're not living the rest of your life right now. You are living today right now. A small part of today, even. This afternoon, this hour, this minute, this second. Right now is the only time you have to deal with. If you deal with all the right now times as best you can, the rest of your life will take care of itself.

...Comparing your losses with someone else's and getting upset because you're behind. I mean, okay I get that we all want it yesterday, but you didn't get here overnight, so the trip back isn't going to be magically short, either. I don't give a rat's booty what anybody else's pace is. It has nothing to do with me. I lose at the rate I lose, and that's fine. Yes, I know it's totally human nature to do this, but it doesn't help.

...Getting disgusted with yourself every time you make a questionable food choice. Yeah, well, you know what? If I judged myself as a total screw-up on the basis of one questionable choice...well gee.

I'd have declared myself a lost cause before I hit my teen years. The trick is making sure helpful choices outnumber and outweigh setback choices. If you expect perfection, you guarantee failure by definition. If you expect progress, you can make progress.

...Waiting for the right configuration of perfect conditions to begin your work. Guess what? The only perfect time is now. There is no time in my life that doesn't have responsibilities, demands, issues. If I waited for these to go away, I'd die first.

...Letting other people make your decisions. Your life is not up for majority rule. If other people pressure you to eat food that's problematic for you, ignore them, pop off a snappy comeback, or promptly burst into tears if you have to; bet they wouldn't do that again soon! So what if people don't approve of your menu? What does that have to do with the price of tea in China? If they're not helping, ignore 'em and cut them out of your personal decision-making loop. They haven't solved your weight problem for you, so what good is shooting down your solution? Just keep moving on and minimize conflict with unhelpful people.

...Maintaining a perfectionist's attitude. If you think you have screwed up the whole day when you take a nibble of a cinnamon roll, well...tossing in the towel for the rest of the day does WAY more damage than the nibbles. What's more helpful for you in the long run: Returning to old, unhealthy habits of gorging yourself with the smallest excuse, or accepting your choices and moving on?

...Sneaking food. This is one of those little, weird things about being overweight. You feel compelled to do your worst eating out of other people's sight. There's almost a feeling if nobody else sees, it doesn't count. Sorry, but I've got bad news. Even if nobody else sees, your ass always knows.

...Not taking care of yourself. If you don't take time to recharge your batteries, relax, refresh yourself, you're operating at a huge disadvantage. Despite all my "Suck it up, Sparky" brand of advice, I know very well that losing weight is challenging. If it were easy, nobody would be fat, 'cause being fat sucks! If you're well-rested, relaxed and happy, it's much easier to make solid, helpful choices.

...Testing your resolve. Why? But people do this all the time. This isn't some kind of sadistic "character test" to see if you can stoically refuse chocolate, for goodness sakes! So be kind to yourself. Do everything you can to make it easier on you. Get the chocolate out of the house if it's a weakness for you, even if the kids whine. It's not negotiable and frankly, it would probably do 'em good if they ate a little less junk anyway, right?

...Burning yourself out. if you think you have to lose 75 pounds overnight and you decide to eat no carbs and exercise 6 hours a day, how long do you think that's gonna last? Learn to look towards moderation. It's a lack of moderation that got your behind in the state it's in now, maybe? So stop using the same overkill hammer on every nail, and try a different approach for a change.

...Loathing yourself as you are. Efforts borne of self-hatred are doomed from the get go. The only reason to improve, to give yourself better, is feeling like you need and deserve better. I'm not saying you have to love the tonnage. Heck no! But...YOU are NOT your fat. Your weight does not define you. Just like you are not your hair color or your eyes or your nose or your clothes or your car or anything else. I think there's more to you than that, don't you? I hope so!

It's not all that hard, really. You get clear on what you are doing and why. You learn how to do it. You take care of yourself as best you can and try to make choices in line with your long-term goals. You stay focused on the long haul.

You may lose a few battles, but you'll win the war.

CHAPTER 17

Guilt Free Dieting

Guilt. It's pervasive in the life of a many a person looking to lose weight.

Guilt over what you've eaten. Guilt over what you didn't eat. (Are you wasting food? Don't you remember those starving children in China?) Guilt over skipping exercise. Even guilt over "wasting" the last how-many-ever years of your life by not watching your weight. If only you had been more vigilant sooner, you wouldn't be in this situation.

Guilt, guilt, guilt! All that guilt is enough to make you fat. Really.

Now as far as I'm concerned, guilt is one of the most useless emotions there is. Guilt is all about living the in the past. It's about feeling bad over something you cannot control. By its very nature, guilt tends to debilitate by moving the focus from NOW–where you have some power to impact your destiny—to then: a place where you can only replay unhappy scenarios that make you feel inferior and ineffective.

I'm not saying that you should never evaluate direction and make changes. I mean, duh. You ignore your own history, you will be repeating it. Correcting course brings you closer to your goals. Of course that has to be done, if you want to make progress.

What I'm saying is way more simple: stop feeling bad that you haven't already reached your goals! That's just silly.

When you play your guilt tapes, what do you hear?

"I'm not good enough. I'm not strong enough. I messed up. I'm just hopeless. I don't have what it takes."

You pound it over and over in your head: I can't make it! Your brain starts to believe, you can't make it. You reinforce an image of yourself as unable to succeed. Over and over and over again, you tell yourself you just don't have the right stuff.

How in the name of God's Green Earth do you expect this kind of nonsense to be helpful? You are simply sending your subconscious the message loud and clear: you don't have what it takes. It's a huge amount of struggle to even tread water. It takes fight, fight, fight to break even. This is deadly to the reach for improvement. You're convincing yourself you aren't even capable of it without even trying!

I'm suggesting something maybe a little radical, especially if you're one of those folks who posts your fat pictures on the refrigerator as motivation—let go of the guilt. When you camp out in the past, you sign off all of your power. You put yourself in a negative, can't-do frame of mind. You give yourself mental pictures of failure, which you replay over and over and over again.

What's the point of that?

Fact is, none of us seem to pop out of the womb fully developed emotionally. And you know what? I wouldn't want to. Life isn't about attaining perfection. It's about the journey. The journey is actually what you have.

The goals? They're just checkpoints along the way. A place to slow down, take a deep breath, and appreciate. If you think about it and you discounted the journey, what would you have left? Milestones and death? I dunno. But I do know I live almost all of my life in the journey. If I don't get my satisfaction from the journey, I'm going to be pretty darned unhappy 99% of the time. I am not into unhappiness.

Much as I love the feeling of reaching a goal, the very reason it's sweet is because it's an accomplishment, a stretch. I worked for it. I am the beneficiary of my experiences–both where I went right and where I went wrong–which I can also share with others, to help them along the way, perhaps. I feel good about it because I learned and grew and worked to get there.

People who are guilt-oriented (and often believe that motivating oneself comes from stronger, sterner castigations) are in for a difficult struggle. The journey? It's a list of your failings, replayed over and over and over. Ow. That approach would make me want to throw my hands up, declare the situation hopeless to stop the pain, and pretend the whole thing never happened. I simply can't imagine how filling your brain with disgust and self-loathing could ever become lasting motivation for self-improvement.

It's true, sometimes an incident, a comment, a situation or a photo may serve as a somewhat rude wakeup call. Smack! "Oh...I didn't know I looked like that in my bathing suit. Eeek! This weight thing is way out of control."

This is good, insofar as you cannot address that which you have not acknowledged. It hurts for a minute, but it makes you aware, in the present! Our layers of denial can be tough to penetrate, and sometimes the Universe has to smack you to get your attention. Okay, I can go along with that.

But once your attention is focused on dealing with your weight and health, then what? Do you root yourself in the past and the (completely irrelevant) question of how you let yourself get there to begin with? Or do you use this realization in the NOW, to learn about your path and make the changes you need to make?

The vibes you put out return to you. You see it in action all the time. The rich get richer, right? Negative people have negative friends, and negative situations abound in their lives. What you believe about yourself and your world is reinforced with your behavior repeatedly and thus, your reality.

In the weight context: If you believe yourself to be weak, undisciplined, unsuccessful and unmotivated, I can promise you without hesitation that is EXACTLY what you will experience. If you call yourself fat, lazy, and gluttonous, that is exactly what you will become. After all, if you believe you just stink at a task, you tend to avoid it. If you feel like you're really moving forward and are getting a payoff for your work, it becomes more exciting and you want to continue.

I don't know why people fail to acknowledge this issue in the context of self-assessment. Perhaps it has to do with internalizing some of society's harsh judgments regarding overweight people. Expand the thought a little bit, and you'll see the truth.

Loving parents seem to understand this approach instinctively. You don't label a child as stupid, lazy, incompetent or unsuccessful, regardless of any momentary difficulty—or even not-so-momentary difficulty. That doesn't help. It only gives the issues root in the child's self-concept and guarantees long-term struggles. You praise the child's efforts. You focus on successes and build on them. You acknowledge progress, focus on progress, and help the child feel successful and happy about progress. Then, you'll continue to see progress.

We've all got a vulnerable part of ourselves that need nurturing, every bit as much as any child ever did.

Are you giving your self-image a black eye with guilt?

Here's what I want you to do: Reframe the past as an incredibly valuable learning experience. That's the true power of past issues: information for future success! If you've been overweight 5 months, 5 years, or 50 years, doesn't matter. You can learn. You can USE your experiences to build upon for future success. You know that parties are tough times for you to manage your eating? Well, plan out alternatives, for goodness sakes! Rather than feeling guilty over that huge lunch out with your coworkers, ask yourself, "What could I do differently next time, to make it easier?"

It's not about stoicism, folks. There is not some bizarre sort of point system where you get moral extra-credit by making things harder on yourself. Guilt does not equal "getting real" or "getting serious" or any other such noteworthy endeavors. Guilt equals punishment.

If you struggle with your weight, you already have experienced the consequences. You have already experienced the pain, the emotional fallout, the limitations, and hit to your self-esteem that comes from being overweight.

Why people sometimes choose to continue slapping themselves when they are already hurting, I have no clue. I think the natural consequences of excess weight are plenty enough. I am not big on punishment, self or otherwise. People don't make good choices out of fear of punishment–or if they do, those choices are hardly internalized. Good choices come from wanting to make good choices, and wanting to experience the consequences of those good choices.

Self-improvement takes work. It takes time to adjust your thinking. It can be uncomfortable to change ingrained habits. In order to maintain the energy and focus to carry you through, believing you can do it helps tremendously. Feeling good about yourself helps tremendously. If ever you are tempted to give up, caring about yourself, loving yourself, and wanting to make the best choices possible for yourself is what will get you through to the other side and ultimate success. Not force-feeding yourself guilt.

You know what? I've tried it both ways. I have had exercise sessions as a perverse sort of punishment for poor eating choices, or even thought of it as just what I got. As a kind of fat penance or something. You have any idea how much that sucks? (Probably yes.) And hey, it's not too hard to guess: punishing yourself doesn't go far towards developing a love of exercise, or the other good habits you will need to adopt for long-term success.

I'm not saying you have to be proud of every decision you've ever made. We're human, and there are times when we look back and wince. That's OKAY.

But now you know what's down that road, you can mark it on your map. You'll know next time, it doesn't go where you want to go (and it probably didn't satisfy the drive that caused you to take that direction anyway).

When you feel you've made a mistake in any area of your life, OKAY. Acknowledge it. See what the experience has to tell you. But then, for God's sakes, move on! Don't sit and wallow in it. Make whatever amends you feel are appropriate–but don't go nuts. Start by considering what you'd expect from your dearest friend in a similar situation. We are so much more loving towards our friends than ourselves, usually.

Every mistake, every wrong turn, every issue we struggle with serves one ultimate purpose: to inform us of areas for progress and growth. That's it.

Every potential guilt trigger is actually a golden opportunity to move ahead. You are being handed a point-by-point primer for success when you experience setbacks of any kind. Frankly, you have a better opportunity for success than the person we may consider lucky, who's had very few setbacks. If you haven't learned your hot-spots and how to rise above and beyond, you get totally thrown when you do hit the inevitable roadblock.

On the other hand, if you've studied your mistakes– just long enough to extract the needed information, mind you–then you know exactly how to proceed. You know you can weather a storm and have important reminders of what is helpful to you, and what is not helpful.

If you can learn to transmute potentially guilty situations into success class, then there really is no stopping you. You know that, right?

Let your slips serve as an education. Me? I have a PhD in how to be fat! But that's not a bad thing.

Because if I clearly understand how I got and stayed fat, I also understand how to avoid it. Reviewing past missteps without self-denigration, I can remain objective enough to extract the lessons there. I know I created that reality, and that's fine. I'm glad I've had the experience set I've had. It's part of who I am.

And the big bonus for me: having had gone through Fat School, I'm now able to share some of my experiences to help others. That makes the pain and struggle that I experienced count for more.

And that boggles my mind sometimes. How cool, you know? Yes, I had those experiences and lived as a fat person. And now, I can make those experiences worthwhile not just to me, but to others who are hurting. What a wonderful gift those mistakes have given me!

Forget the guilt, man! It's a beautiful journey, if you are open to seeing it.

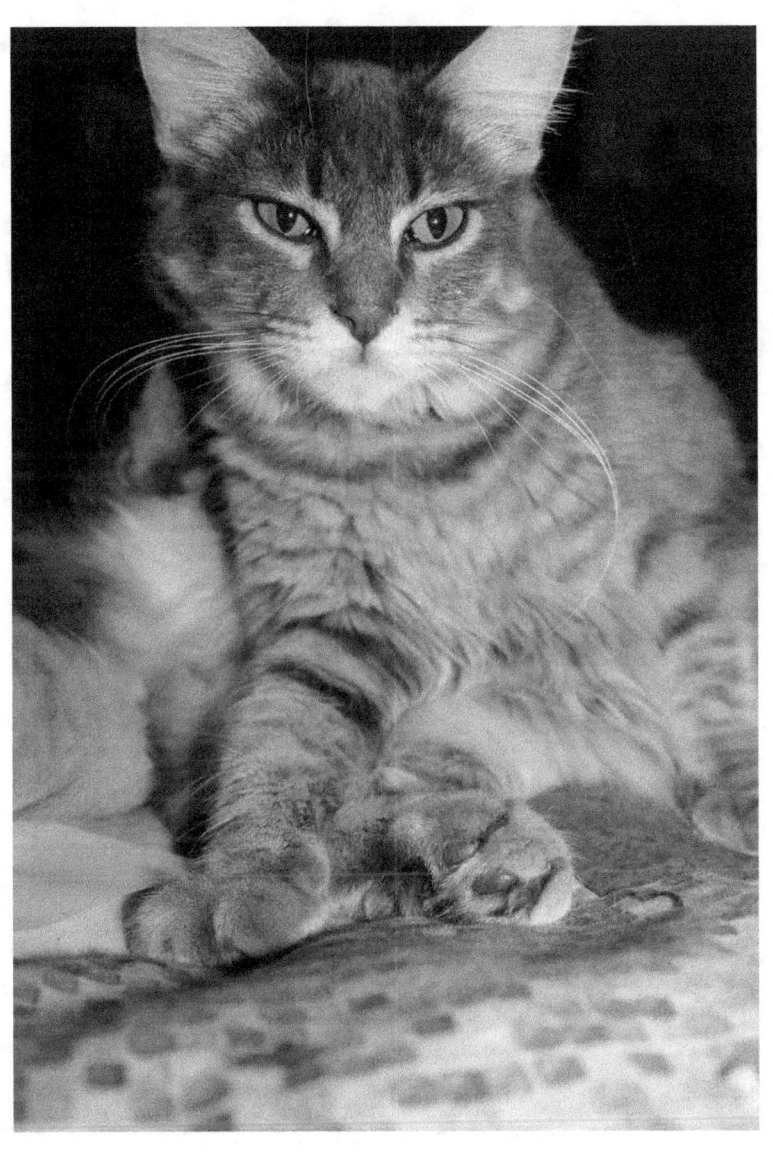

Attitude Adjustments

CHAPTER 18

A Losing Attitude

One of the best indicators of successful weight loss I've found in the trenches is not diet plan, amount of weight to lose, age, medical concerns, or any of the other, usual suspects.

It's WAY more simple. I'll give you a hint: Attitude.

My self-esteem was basically intact pushing 300 pounds, but I didn't feel good about that part of my life. Mostly, I'd just relegate it to my subconscious, out of my view. I didn't like my appearance, so I told myself that it "wasn't that bad." I told myself it was just too difficult to lose weight, not worth the effort.

Who cares about all that superficial stuff, right?

But I did care. I tried very hard not to care, but I never stopped caring.

So a harsh self-assessment and self-recrimination is NOT an effective tool for weight loss. How could it be?

Have you met many seriously overweight people who haven't spent a significant chunk of time telling themselves how much they suck? I know this is not true universally, but I came up way before the body positivity movement, man.

Yes, okay, sometimes it may be feelings of self-disgust that provide an initial kick-in-the-pants to get started. Maybe you've been in denial. I have my own condo in the state of denial, thank you very much.

And okay, if it gets you started, then it's helpful—maybe we need a jolt to be shocked out of sugar-induced complacency or something.

But just looking at the sheer numbers of people who are both overweight and hate themselves for it—well, it's obvious the harsh self-assessments are not a prescription for success. In fact, if you're fat, you may well try to eat your way out of bad feelings.

We eat in part to deal with stress, boredom, anxiety, sadness, or anger. You name it, we can eat it right up. Looking to numb pain? Food works. And assessing oneself as "disgusting, lazy, sloppy, gluttonous," or whatever other insults you hurl is pain, no?

So, you have the initial pain that sent you to the kitchen. You have the pain from the physical consequences from overeating. And you have the pain from the negative self-assessment. Ugh. It's a viciously circular pain-fest, man.

If you are coming from a place of self-disgust and you slip a bit—well, there goes the negative barrage, right? You tell yourself you're lazy and weak and a screw-up and/or whatever your own hot spot accusations. Hence, that slip leads to the negative internal dialog, which leads to you feeling crummier, which leads to you wanting to numb that pain the way you've numbed pain for years, most likely—sugary, sweet, carb-packed comfort food!

Not to mention that fact that each time you go through this cycle, you also reinforce that inner programming, that the goal of achieving a comfortable and healthy body weight is beyond your capacity to achieve. NOT good!

Pure and simple: You get what you focus on. How can you even imagine that telling yourself over and over that you're lazy, stupid, weak-willed and a screw-up would produce anything but exactly those results? You become who the tapes in your head say you are!

Why not reprogram the tapes? Why not let those tapes say that you're strong, you're talented, you're smart, and you're worthy?

I'm not trying to be Stuart Smalley. The thing is, each time you say kind things to yourself, you'll believe it a little more. As you come to believe it more, you come to act in concert with those beliefs.

If you feel crummy about yourself, then it's easy to feel like you deserve to remain fat. It becomes inevitable punishment for your perceived flaws. If you feel good about yourself on the other hand, then you can believe you deserve to be well taken care of and healthy.

Now, I'm not saying this is always easy. You've probably got years of the self-effacing messages to overcome. Most of us do. But overcome you can, if you want to, if you choose to. When you hear one of those negative messages in your head, stop yourself immediately and correct it!

"No, wait. I'm not weak or lazy. I made a choice that didn't support my long-term goals. That's it. I don't think it was worth it. Next time, I'll make a different choice."

See how much easier that is?

Believing that you deserve to be healthy and happy is going to carry you through lots of potential pitfalls. You think you deserve that chocolate cake? I think you deserve to feel good and be healthier!

You think of yourself as lazy? Well, if you start thinking of yourself as becoming stronger every day, it becomes a lot easier to go ahead and do some exercise. Then, you're not fighting the tide any more. You're transforming.

Changing ain't easy. You'll find, though, once you work on your thinking, the life-changing action bits fall right into place. When the situations come up— and they will—where you're faced with challenging decisions, coming from a positive place, you make positive decisions. Sure, maybe not everything in the world has lined up to your expectations. But you're working on it, right? And you are getting closer every day, should you choose to do so.

We ARE the creators of our lives. Our thoughts are a form of energy that goes out into the Universe, you know? Thoughts are the equivalent of silent prayers, especially repeated over and over.

If you repeatedly tell yourself you're a victim, you're going to find perpetrators. If you believe you're weak, you're attracting incidents that reinforce weakness. And if you believe that you're a lazy, undisciplined, hopeless case—well, I think you know where this is going.

But you know the alternative already. People say, "You are what you eat." That's not exactly right. It's more like you are what you THINK you are. What you eat is incidental to who you are.

But what you eat can deplete or enhance your life force, the energy budget you have to live out what you think you are.

So just be kind to yourself, okay? The world needs you and your gifts. Your loved ones need you and your gifts.

You can do this. So do!

CHAPTER 19

Fat Pix as a Deterrent?

Now, I don't respect you any less if this is what you do. This is just how I feel about it, okay? Everybody has to find their own path, I know. That having been said, though...

I've heard people mention keeping fat pictures, on the fridge or in their wallets or something. As a deterrent for cheating, y'kno. As a reminder of how disgusting they find themselves fat, a sort of smack to keep them on the straight and narrow. Except...well, when I hear such things, I just feel sad.

I mean, gosh. I was NOT unworthy when I was fat. I wasn't lazy or immoral or stupid or ugly. I was just fat. I liked chocolate too much, for God's sake.

I'm not saying that being fat was good for me. It wasn't. Actually, it got in my way. My body had aches, pains, and physical discomfort. I had less energy and stamina, so I didn't accomplish as much as I might. I did not feel as good about myself as I could have.

I've been fat and I've been not fat, and I WAY prefer not fat. It's completely worth the effort! But let's take a little closer look at these attitudes, shall we?

I'm not saying I thought it was cool when I noticed in a picture that I was considerably fatter than I realized in my head. Heck no! That sucks. It did help me realize how much the issue was getting out of hand. But that's the only real function it served.

And now when I look at my fat pictures? They make me feel really good. They remind me of how much I've accomplished! I feel good about the weight I lost, not because I was less than complete before. I was fine before. But losing the weight was a significant accomplishment that I'm proud of. It's healthier for me and more fun to be skinnier. It gives me joy, so it was a good thing.

See, I am beautiful now, but I was beautiful then, too. I had love in my life, both then and now. I see beauty in love, that's the most beautiful thing in the world to me. Beauty doesn't come from your physical body. It's not in the shape of your nose or what size clothes you wear. I am beautiful because of the love I have in my heart, the joy I take in life, helping and connecting with others, That's where true, permanent beauty comes from.

Beauty has absolutely nothing to do with the size of your jeans. In fact, I can't think of a LESS meaningful measurement of beauty. You can be beautiful at any age and any weight, for God's sakes. You just have to let the light of who you really are shine out authentically to be beautiful. And for that, the outside stuff doesn't matter.

Now, I do think losing weight makes this easier. You have more energy to share and you spend less time hiding. Your confidence grows and you're more likely to risk letting yourself be honestly seen. But it doesn't mean you were less-than, before.

Yes, I much prefer how I look and feel physically, now. But it's a bonus, not a prerequisite to being an acceptable human being.

So why tear yourself down, telling yourself over and over what a disgusting creature you are? That won't make you skinnier, or more beautiful, or happier or better in any way, I promise you. Good things always come from good places in your heart.

You become what you believe yourself to be. I don't know about you, but I'm choosing to be beautiful!

CHAPTER 20

Fatbutt Syndrome

I don't mean to be flip...well, maybe I do. I'll cop. But that's the million dollar question, 'eh? Maybe it's the billion dollar question, what with the diet industry being what it is. How do we get to be fatbutts, and what does one do about it?

And don't even start babbling to me about calories! You're liable to get slapped where you stand. I get flat-out angry when I hear the old calories-in-versus-calories-out-routine:

"It's a simple matter of calories in versus calories out. You eat less and exercise more, and you will lose weight."

Implied argument? Stop being such a stupid, lazy, greedy pig, and you'll cease to be fat.

Yeah. Thanks for the newsflash, huh? Without that amazing insight, it never would have occurred to us to eat less and exercise more, huh?

Geez.

Aside: Extremely low-calorie diets and lots of strenuous exercise—in other words, the purportedly complete and infallible calories-in-vs.-calories-out formula taken too extremes—will cause your body to cannibalize muscles for the protein it requires to survive. Ummm.. This is NOT exactly healthy. Bonus penalty: Muscle is approximately 8 times denser than fat, and it burns more of those hated calories than fat, even at a resting state. This is also why new exercisers don't always immediately see results on the scale, even while their pants are falling off. Love your muscles and they will love you. Treat your muscles as well as you'd treat your dog. Feed them, water them, and take them for regular walks. They will thank you for it with smaller sizes and more energy. But if you're overweight, you probably already know most of this. Stop living and dying by that evil little machine, and listen to your body, 'K Sparky? End aside.

That goes to show you how little most people get it. Have you ever met an overweight person past puberty who hasn't tried dozens upon dozens of diets? I mean anything and everything: fasting, living on grapefruit, cabbage soup, the rice diet (and those little Styrofoam rice cakes taste as nasty as they look), countless supplements, prescription drugs, nothing but salad for days on end, chugging SlimFast, popping Dexatrim like candy, or worse yet, actually drinking TAB?

Shudder.

Ask any random fattie, and s/he will be able to tell you almost anything you want to know about dieting. A fat person's knowledge of dieting would put most professionals to shame! They will know calories, carbs or fat counts of half the contents of the neighborhood grocery store without blinking. They know the name of the various weight-loss drugs and supplements and how they work. They can off-handedly tell you who is a candidate for gastric bypass, who is not, and why. They've read and studied and pondered every little morsel of weight loss information known to mankind, usually more than once.

So why are so many of us still fat?

Diets. Don't. Work. Are you listening? DIETS DON'T WORK!

Dieting as a concept reminds me of what Mark Twain said about smoking. "Giving up smoking is the easiest thing in the world. I know because I've done it thousands of times."

He's right. In this case, the problem is not losing the weight. Not even close.

Here's what happens. Fat person feels it's time to "suck it up and deal with the weight." This often is prompted by something like an unflattering photograph, or maybe a trip to the doctor, or aches and pains or whatever. Doesn't matter. Something starts the weight-loss train in motion by creating pain in fat person's life.

Fat person starts to feel guilty for being fat to begin with. "I'm so lazy. I have no willpower. I'm such a pig. Why do I eat all this anyway?" Fat person feels like crap.

Fat person either beings to drown sorrows in a vat of Ben & Jerry's or, at least for a while, begins to punish his or her fat self by existing on a few blades of grass each day coupled with an exercise plan that would make a squirrel on meth collapse.

And like every effort born out of self-loathing, it is doomed to fail. We have this annoying little function built into our brains called "a survival instinct." So unlike alcoholics who decide to leave the booze behind, we can't stop eating. (And unlike recovering Alcoholics, who usually have social support for their efforts, we have those coworkers, friends or family elbowing us in the ribs and insisting, "Just a little bit won't hurt you.")

And while we're at it...we are not enjoying the exercise frenzy—it's hard work to exercise when you're overweight! Particularly when you first start, it can be especially exhausting and difficult. You may feel embarrassed of your appearance, frustrated at how much energy it all takes, disturbed you don't have more stamina, and angry at yourself for being here in the first place. And God help you if you've ate some cake that you're punishing yourself for via the stair climber.

Whew! Am I hitting pay dirt here? Been there more times than I can count, man.

Doesn't exactly sound like the perfect setup for success, huh? Even those of us who are overweight usually want to like ourselves. We get sick of obsessing or worse, feeling guilty for every little bite of food that passes our lips, "legal" or not. That's what it's like, you know. Sooner or later, most fat people start to hate themselves with every single bite.

We're tired, we're hungry, and we're sore from that &*&^$ elliptical trainer. Work sucked and those cookies look mighty comforting. So we say, "Screw it." Either we declare ourselves hopeless and unable to make the changes needed, or we try to convince ourselves we don't care, although we still do, because not caring is much less painful that hating yourself. And you might even feel better, for a few minutes.

But there you are, right where you started, except your already battered self-esteem has taken a few more blows. And your knees still hurt, too.

Ouch.

Overweight people do NOT need to learn about losing weight, since almost all of us already know that subject intimately. We cuss and cajole ourselves for not being strong enough, and condemn ourselves because our efforts don't pay off quickly enough. It must be that we're still too lazy to exercise "enough," or still too weak to cut down those stupid calories "enough" or still lacking willpower because we are hungry and tired on those 1000 calories a day or yada, yada, yada.

The underlying theme here is repeatedly telling ourselves we are not good enough. To which I say: Bull hockey.

We need to feel good about ourselves. Feeling bad is fattening. And being in a big, fat hurry to lose the big, fat belly isn't helping.

So what the answer?

See, the problem isn't figuring out how to go about losing weight. Overweight people are already bloody experts on the topic, okay? It's finding what works permanently that's the real issue here.

It's not about cutting down the girth as quickly as possible. While fast losses are more fun than a more measured approach, crash dieting doesn't teach you what you have to learn to be free from this albatross forever. Keeping the *$(%* weight off is hard part!

Can I get an Amen, brothers and sisters?

Love thyself. That's what it all boils down to. I keep hammering on this, but there are still a few folks who haven't seen the light.

Losing weight is an act of self-love. It may have been the pain that got your attention, but working on your weight is protecting your health and well-being and therefore, by definition is taking care of yourself. (Perk: You have more energy to care for others and you set a good example for your kids and loved ones. Double-perk: It will drive the ex insane. Har!)

There are many ways of taking care of yourself. But one thing I can say without reservation. While specific changes may be challenging at first, taking care of yourself does not involve being mean to yourself. So forget self-denigration, excessive deprivation, or crazed exercise frenzies that leave you frustrated and depressed. I mean, c'mon. That's never worked before has it?

How are you successful without all the pain? Here's the trick. Stop focusing on losing the weight, and start focusing on improving your habits. Don't think that you won't lose weight that way, because you will. Take care of today's choices, and tomorrow will automatically materialize better than yesterday.

We need easy, comfortable ways to fit weight-loss goals into our everyday lives. We have to learn ways to lose weight that don't make us feel frustrated, deprived, and less of a person for having weight to lose in the first place. We need to find exercise that is enjoyable and helps us feel a sense of joy, accomplishment and mastery, not like ungraceful cows, you know?

So how do you do that?

Tips on Eliminating the FatButt Syndrome:

Take a Pollyanna Challenge. Eliminate all negative self-talk right out of the chute. This step alone will help you start feeling better and more optimistic. It won't happen unless you at least concede it as a possibility, man, and that negative self-talk will kick your butt in that regard. If you have trouble with this step, whenever you start to rag on yourself, imagine you are talking to a friend instead—someone you care for deeply. We would never talk to friends in the crummy ways we talk to ourselves.

Make a change. What? You thought I would excuse you from the work? Fat chance, friend. Snort! But here's the deal. Make this a small, relatively painless change to start. Now, I am not going to insult your intelligence by telling you to put your fork down between bites of food or something. This is not a sidebar in a women's magazine, dude. And that crap makes me want to slap people, when it's presented like some sort of magic formula. But maybe you can cut down on sugar intake (or cut it out, if you're already moving in that direction), up your water or dance after dinner. Whatever seems helpful and is the easiest and most pleasant for you, do that first. Then build on it.

Focus on habits, not individual events. In the grand scheme, one event doesn't matter either way. It's the habits, the choices you make most consistently day in and day out that will determine your level of success.

Feel good and celebrate your successes. Another pointer? No fattening, sugar-encrusted, chocolate-covered celebrations for losing weight, Sparkster. It is counter-productive. But do celebrate and acknowledge your progress, even if it's nothing more than just taking a minute to feel good about what you've done. This is vital. Success is the most motivating feeling in existence.

Don't say you've been "good" or "bad" based on food choices. That's all hogwash, okay? Eating is not a moral issue. You can tell me you feel good about the choices you've been making, and that's great. But you're not a two-year old getting a behavior report from daycare already. For the better days, congratulate yourself and move on. For the rougher days, ask yourself what you might change next time, and move on. You have inherent worth for being you. So lighten up already!

Incorporate exercise, but reasonably. What does that mean? Well, if the most exercise you've gotten in the last decade is running to the bathroom when you get home after being stuck in traffic, take it slow. And for goodness sakes, don't pick your exercise based on what's the most intense or burns the most calories. Do what you like! If you hate it, you'll be miserable doing it. If it's fun for you, then after the initial resistance to starting any exercise program, you will find yourself doing it because you like to do it, and you like the feeling it gives you. People who keep that weight off exercise, and you want to be in the group, don't ya? Do a little at first, and then a little more, and then a little more. Take your time. If you like trees, walk in the park. If you like music, dance. If you like scenery, take up biking. But whatever you do, just do something!

Rinse and repeat. Build on each step, and move on to the next. I'm not saying not to push your comfort zone here. You have to! Change can be challenging, and we're talking about deeply ingrained behaviors undergoing revision, I know. But poke on that envelope gradually, gently, in a way that leaves you feeling strong and powerful. In other words, yes, you can challenge yourself so long as it feels good, but make sure the challenges are moderate and ongoing.

Pat yourself on the back and enjoy your progress. And progress not just a number on the evil little scale, either. Progress is feeling better. Progress is having more energy. Progress is your tight jeans feeling more comfortable. Progress is making healthy choices and feeling good about it. Progress is leaving the obsession behind you, and feeling in control of your weight and your life.

Finally, NEVER surrender. There is only one true way to fail, and it's to give up! If you're still here, you're still in the game. So keep putting one foot in front of the other. Take care of today, now, right this minute and the future will be there for you, all pretty like, without any special intervention on your part. Funny how that works.

There is no rush. There is no fire to be put out. You go back to your old habits, you go back to your old pants size, plain and simple. So understand this is for life. And since it is for life, it needs to be a life you can be happy with and live comfortably in, long-term.

Yes, you have to make changes to lose weight. Duh. But make manageable and consistent changes, and you will progress without all the pain. Be the tortoise, and let the hare burn himself out by January 8th. You? You're just out taking a walk after dinner, and you feel great doing it.

I will put my money on the people that consistently make small, helpful changes they feel good about over the master dieter who knows how to crack that whip on himself any day.

Feed your head with positive energy and it will pay off. It's not as hard as it looks. And you will be so glad you did. That's a promise.

Be good to yourselves out there!

CHAPTER 21

Feeling Bad is Fattening

People, having fallen off the wagon, commonly get mired in predictable lines of thinking.

Aside: Why do we call it "falling off the wagon" anywho? Like we're all riding along on a big, happy, low-carb wagon and just having a grand ol' time. Whhhhooooa...bump in the road. Traffic ticket! Or spouse got the flu, or the car broke down. Bump! The wagon jars and off you plop!

When you sit around having your little pity party– and I'm not judging, because I've been there, man– but when you settle in, upset and throwing around thoughts of deprivation and how you can "never manage to be good, blah, blah, blah, ad infinitum?" Well, where do you think that leads?

[Ba-da-bum!] The fridge, of course.

You're feeling bad about yourself, questioning your ability to even do this, thinking "there's no point." Self-define as a failure and follow up with self-fulfilling prophecy. Wrapped up tight, with a big, sad bow, that's the whole package.

If, HOWEVER, you want to really do something with it, start by saying, "So what?"

So what? The past is done.

THIS moment, this very second, is the only point in time we have any real power. The future is imagination and the past, memory. There is only now.

Even if your thoughts are positive, if they are firmly rooted within the past or the future, you're not ACTING in the present. One action does more in the physical world than a billion and two thoughts. I know. I've thought the billion and two thoughts.

Don't get me wrong. I consider thoughts to have real, energetic weight. But we must use our energy to guide us in the physical world. One of the most important functions of managing our thinking is to drive ACTION.

The difference between feeling bad and feeling good is probably 97% interpretation. It's all in how you frame it, baby. And the same goes for a slide. You can either define it as proof positive that you aren't cut out to be successful OR you can define it as a short break, a learning experience to help you grow and hence, be in a better position to ultimately reach your goal.

See, it doesn't matter jack squat how FAST you go. People think it does and get all whiney. Myself included. But if this is just how you live, then what's a week here or there? I don't give a %$^* in *&% ^@% how long it takes. Totally irrelevant. The ONLY thing that's relevant is that you're doing what you need to do NOW.

Being in a hurry implies that you are someday done. You go back to your old way of eating, you'll go back to your old diameter. That's clear. And while I agree that there's some psychological appeal to goals and milestones, they aren't the actual progress. They are simply markers, reminders. Opportunities to reflect and appreciate.

And here's the real kicker–if you're eating crap that you don't feel good about eating, you don't enjoy it much anyway. You feel guilty and unhappy the entire time. But that sure as heck doesn't stop the downslide! In fact, what do we do? We eat MORE of the same crap in an attempt to self-medicate the distress we get from eating the crap in the first place.

Man, that makes my hair hurt if I think about it too hard.

I have never, ever met somebody who truly enjoyed more than the first 3 bites of a binge. Have you? After bite three, I'm starting to feel so down on myself, it's not tasting very good anymore.

But you know how it works: keep shoveling it in long enough, you have to feel better eventually. Right? Right?!

Well...maybe not.

You get what you focus on. You think about it, you visualize it, you live it. That's how the universe works. So when you're feeling bad about how you're doing, answer me this. What are you focusing on?

Are you thinking about how fat and unhappy and weak and lazy and just plain "bad" you are? That sounds like the recipe for success right there...NOT.

But if you're focusing on how much better you feel when you eat right, how you've made progress here and there, and overall how life's going well enough (even if you have to dig a little for the "well enough"), those thoughts confer energy, motivation, momentum. Unlike feeling crappy, which sends you diving into a vat of Ben & Jerry's without even a few carb-blockers to break your fall.

Reality isn't contained solely in events themselves; reality exists in tandem with our interpretation of those events. Remember that.

Feeling good energizes you, motivates you, helps you sleep at night and work and play well with others. And I wouldn't be surprised if it doesn't make your teeth whiter and your hair shinier, for that matter. Whereas feeling bad sucks and it doesn't help you in any way, shape or form... so just don't do it, okay?

Ditch the crap and get back to living the way it feels best.

No remorse, just lessons. Okay? Just lessons.

CHAPTER 22

Feeling Skinny is Fun (& Builds Success)

The skinnier you feel, the less you're interested in temptation.

Losing weight means your self-image is in flux, and it's sometimes hard to match how your body is changing to how you feel. It's can be disorienting,

But feeling good helps keep us on track, so feeling good is incredibly important. To do your best, it's vital to maximize positive energy.

No matter where you are on your journey, it's not hard to make slight adjustments in your behavior and thinking that help you feel skinnier, and therefore more motivated.

And to top that off, it's fun, too! Seriously. Try it for a while, and I think you'll agree it's WAY better than feeling fat! Also? Not so hard. I'll tell you how to do it.

Have lots of ways to measure progress. Clothing fit, tape measure, BMI changes, journals, energy, activity levels, etc. The idea is that you maintain a sense of success totally separate from what the scale says.

Keep slightly snug clothing stashed to try on regularly. Obviously, this shouldn't be your whole wardrobe. But you will regularly surprise yourself by fitting easily into something you didn't know you could.

Always have a few outfits that fit just right and you feel great in! Nothing motivates like success. Bonus: When you wear clothes that fit, you (and others) can see how much weight you've really lost.

Stay hydrated. Keeping up on your water will help you stay on track, plus you'll feel better and your skin will be softer. You don't tend to bloat when you get plenty of H20, and it helps those losses flow.

Forget lose-by dates. If you miss the mark by even a few ounces, you can end up feeling like a failure. Instead, set moderate, behaviorally-based goals that you have control over. Celebrate each step.

Look at old pictures, and take some new ones. When you're losing weight, body image is in an incessant state of flux. It's hard to judge what size clothes you need; some days, you'll feel gloriously thin. Other day, you'll feel like a river barge. Pictures help ground your self-image while your body is in transformation, because you'll need that frame of reference.

Try different styles. Be a little more daring that you usually would. It's fun to be vain and experiment with different styles. You'll find as you go along your old style doesn't fit you anymore, anyway. So find out what does fit you now.

Take your vitamins. Of course, you're eating well. But even so, at least a solid Multivitamin will make sure you're getting what you need and help keep you feeling perky and energetic.

Encourage others. It keeps your vibration high and clear, and gives your brain time focusing on positive, helpful info. Win-win, baby!

Here's wishing you all a very skinny day, and many more of 'em!

CHAPTER 23

Scale-itis

A common dieter's disease that you see running rampant: Scale-itis. As in: How can I lose 2 kajillion pounds in three minutes?

Now I get this. I SO get it. But if you stop for even just a second to think about where it comes from, it may change your perspective a bit.

You've seen people who have EVERY SINGLE indication of being successful at losing weight, short having the scale read what they want, and what happens? Blind panic, right?

"Well, yes, I know I've lost 500 inches and I feel great and I can climb the Matterhorn now and I know that I've gained lots of muscle and I now wear clothes 19 sizes smaller...but I wanna lose WEIGHT! The scaaaaalllllllle! The scale doesn't say the number I want it to say!"

You gotta wonder, why is that one number all that matters?

And after giving it some thought, I think I get it. That number is what they're using as a self-definition, entirely. Forget "you are what you eat." These people are thinking, "I am what I weigh."

While numbers are a convenient way of measuring success, they're not to be mistaken for the ACTUAL success. We use numbers as an easy and quick way to communicate status, a common language that folks can understand and quantify.

But the real goals aren't—or at least shouldn't be—those stupid numbers on a hunk of gears and metal. Numbers which, I may add, will change depending on the time of day, water retention, hormonal cycles, where on the floor the contraption sits, and which way you lean when hopping on the darned thing for your moment of reckoning.

That tiny little scale becomes an evil dictator by which we judge our entire self worth, and it needs to stop! Yes, I know you have your vacation-reunion-birthday-anniversary party coming up in ten minutes now. You think there isn't always some kind of milestone coming up?

I'm as human as the rest of you. You think it doesn't feel good to say, "I've lost a hundred pounds?" Think again. Think I don't get excited to see those numbers falling on the scale along with everybody else? Heck yeah, I do!

But of course, it's never a problem when the numbers are going DOWN, is it? It's only the upward swings that we take panic-stricken notice of.

Nonetheless, those fluctuations ARE part of the process for all of us, like it or not, Sparky. If you weigh yourself regularly, you will see normal fluctuations. Or even not-so-normal fluctuations. Whatever you see, you see. There's no cause for panic (or exercising 4 hours a day or trying to live on 3 lettuce leaves and some nasty ol' TAB, man).

All extreme measures actually do is guarantee that you will not consistently follow through on your half-baked plan to get that scale reading down, long term. If you're concerned about losses moving slowly, how about doing something sensible? You could up your water intake, add some movement, start following an earlier phase of your plan, or even put that scale in a closet for a month while you work on making healthy, obsession-free choices.

Frankly, if you can't see the numbers fluctuate without freaking out, then throw out your bloody scale and get on with your life!

It's sort of like money. You could have all the money in the world, but if you didn't know how to spend it in a way that brought comfort and satisfaction, why bother? Weight loss is similar. It's something you do for your health, or to look better and feel better. And if you're constantly nagging on yourself about how you haven't hit a silly little number...well, you're missing the point in a major way. What about all the progress you've made?

If you are having trouble staying grounded and repeatedly hitting panic mode (which, at least half the time, will progress into binging-mode), stop. Take a minute to remind yourself of the reasons why you decided to do this in the first place. I'll bet you money it wasn't because of a number on a scale. Even if it was a reading on the scale that got your attention, it wasn't the number per se, but the meaning that number has to you. Very different.

Chances are, you started this journey was because you were concerned about your health or your appearance or the example you're setting for your children or any one of a million other reasons. The number has whatever meaning you give it. Once person may feel fat at 125; somebody else may feel thin at 325. It's not the number, folks.

Don't get fixated on any arbitrary measure of success, especially at the expense everything that prompted and fueled the journey thus far. If you feel great, are in control of your eating, and are healthy...well, what difference does it make what the scale has to say about it?

And even if you aren't where you want, scale-wise or otherwise, so what?

Just keep moving in the direction you want to go and you'll get there in due time. Stop complaining about the speed you're going and start enjoying the ride, man.

Life isn't the destination, anyway. It's the trip. So enjoy your trip.

CHAPTER 24

Dressing for Weight Loss Success

No. I'm not talking heavy sweaters! When you're losing weight, many things change. Stuff you used to take for granted changes. Even dressing becomes a much more complicated issue. You thought it was the opposite, didn't you? You have more choices; your clothes aren't too tight anymore.

And that's true, sure. However, there's more to it than that. Actually, the clothing decisions that you make now are sending very specific messages to your brain.

There is a very easy way to "Dress for Success" in this case. The clothes you keep indicate quite clearly what your expectations are about.

Can't bear to get rid of your fat clothes, "just in case?" What message does that send if it's not, "Hey, this weight-loss thing is temporary? I'd better hold on to those fat clothes because I'm going back."

I mean, good lord. What else could this mean? There are so many implications; the messages you're giving yourself are not too helpful.

I don't trust myself to maintain these positive changes.

I'm going to make a nice show of trying before I go back to my old ways.

It won't last. It never does.

I can't make it.

Plain and simple, keeping those fat clothes betray a subconscious decision to stay fat. Sound harsh? I'm sorry, but that's where this leads. You're putting your money where your mouth is, literally.

Which "you" are you the most invested in: the old, fatter you, or the new, skinnier you?

Now, I understand when people are actively losing weight, they put off buying new clothing. I know your budget would probably be happier if you don't buy a completely new wardrobe every time you lose ten pounds. But, it's actually very helpful to have one or two outfits on hand at all times that you feel very good in. They have to fit well and you have to believe them flattering. These can be second-hand, old clothes you haven't been able to wear in a long time or new. It's not as important where they come from as it is what they do for you, you know?

And while we're on the topic: Don't let other people decide what these clothes should be! If you want to dress like a hippie chick, if you want to describe your outfit as "pimpin'," well, okay. That's your choice. The ONLY requirement is that you feel good in the clothes!

Losing weight is a relatively slow process. The gratification is gradual. Things happen a little bit at a time and invariably, there will be moments when you'll feel discouraged. It gets tedious giving so much energy and focus to losing weight sometimes. So, what do you do? You need support staying focused.

If you have a few outfits that you feel like a million bucks wearing, you can remind yourself of all the positive changes you've made. You can see your progress! And there is another perk. When you wear smaller sized clothing that fits, people will notice losses. When you're still swimming along in your 3X shirts and using a belt to keep those baggy pants from sliding off...it hides losses much more efficiently than it hides fat. But when you move on to the proper size for the new you, you look better, you feel better, and you're in the process of learning who that "new you" is.

And I'll go one further. I'd like you to get one more item of clothing the meets two criteria: 1) You'd love wearing it; and 2) It's about a size too small.

Yeah, too small. This is the message you're giving yourself here is, "I'm losing weight, and I'll soon be able to wear this comfortably. I'm looking forward to it!"

Which message do you want to generate? Which reality do you want to create?

So pitch the fat pants! That doesn't have to be literal. I highly recommend donating them, actually. That way, you can feel good about sharing and you get to move on to what's right for you, now. That's smaller clothes, because you're committed to success.

And while you're at it, get a couple of nice outfits for you to wear in your current size, and a thing or two that is too small. Look for sales and other serendipitous wardrobe building opportunities, okay?

Keeping reinforcing what you want to be your reality, and soon it WILL be your reality. Really. Really-really.

Dress for your success. Capitalize on it, revel in it, focus on it, and enjoy it. That's the surest way there is to generate more!

CHAPTER 25

Lose-By Dates: Help or Hindrance?

I know for some folks, having a lose-by date can be motivating and help keep them on track, focused. At least, that's what they tell me. But for many, these dates can often become a bigger obstacle than help.

You may be asking the wrong questions. Instead of "How can I lose this many pounds by this date?" maybe the question should be, "How can I continue to make sustainable progress I can maintain?"

I know, know, know it's so natural to be in a hurry. I started out as one of the worst offenders! You have any idea how many calculations I did of my "done date?" I set up a spreadsheet for it. I had it down to the day. (Short answer is never. You go back to the old ways, you will go back to the old pants-size. But that idea wasn't part of my thinking, early on.)

How many times anything in life go perfectly, with no sidetracks? Frankly, I've almost never seen a lose-by date that takes reality adequately into account.

Besides, why on Earth would it matter if you lose the next 20 pounds by August or December? If you set this goal in stone and then are delayed—either by choices you've made or just how your body decides to do its own thing (and those bodies do)— you're left feeling inadequate, unsuccessful, and discouraged. No matter how well you've done in reality, if you miss some arbitrary lose-by date, in your mind you're screwing it up and your mind runs this show.

What happens in a straight line from point A to point B? My weight GAIN sure wasn't! Surprising, considering the way I used to eat. Part of my journey has been coming to terms with detours on the road. To me, the question is, "What purpose does the rush serve?" Is it helping or hindering?

Fear can be a real issue here. I was TERRIFIED once I started having some real success, my solution would stop working. I had to hurry, lest my magic bullet lost its bite! It was all just a big anomaly, I tell you. Temporary and fleeting. That's certainly how it felt. I was afraid to keep believing. If you believe, you can be disappointed.

But the other side of that coin is, if you believe, you can succeed, too. If you don't have the belief, the first little bump, the first little stall or delay will serve to convince you that this won't work for you or you don't have what it takes. And missing a lose-by goal can serve as the bump.

Eventually, I came to the conclusion that I needed to feel good about the successes I'd already had, and even if I never lost another ounce, I'd done myself wonderful good.

Success can be scary in many ways! You know the status quo. You don't know what happens when you let go of that familiar place, though. I'll tell you one thing. If you have a lot of weight to lose and you lose it, your life WILL change.

But mostly, I was left with the idea that I had to let go of tomorrow and the how-will-I-do-all-this-anyway ideas and when-is-it-gonna-be-done-already questions completely, and just experience today.

I started constructing my goals around making good choices today, right now, right this minute. That, I had control over. I quickly discovered if I took care of NOW, the future has this amazing way of coming together all by itself.

I think being anxious and concerned about the pace of losses is very natural, but not usually helpful. My advice is to accept the fact that you don't have complete control of how your body functions and that does not define you as success or failure.

Instead, just take care of now, and I promise you, the future becomes greater without the any special intervention. Small steps taken at the pace that's right for you will still get you where you're going. Keep taking those steps, one foot after the other.

The rest will come together in due time.

CHAPTER 26

Eliminating Temptation in 1 Easy Step!

I know that's a mighty big promise. And you're not reading a back issue of the *Weekly World News* where the next article is about Bat-boy mating with Alien-chick. Nope. This is a one-step primer for how to totally eliminate all temptation from your life. But before we get rid of it, let's define it.

I saw a quote on the topic that rather struck me.

"If you would not step into the harlot's house, do not go by the harlot's door." -Thomas Secker

If you don't want to eat the cookies, you don't hang near the cookie jar. If you constantly toy with the idea of doing stuff you say you don't want to do, you're still on your way to doing it. I've said it a million times, so now it's a million and one: you get what you focus on!

Don't want to drink? Then don't hang out at the bar, studying the issue. Don't want to pack on a couple of pounds of cookie weight? Then steer clear of the cookie tray, sister (or brother, as the case may be).

And please, don't tell me you "couldn't help yourself." I would have to slap you, and neither of us wants that. You may think I'm kidding, but do you really want to chance it?

The thoughts you feed are the ones that grow. The thoughts you neglect die off eventually. So if you're tired of struggling with a temptation, it's quite easy to remedy.

Starve it. Don't hang out by the Harlot's door if you don't intend to go in. 'Cause if you keep hanging out there...well, sooner or later you're going peek inside. Maybe not today, maybe not even tomorrow, but definitely next week.

In that sense, temptation is a sort of aberration. What we call temptation is nothing more than the period of time that you are toying with an idea. It's not the situation itself, it's the pause in between desire and decision. The time standing outside the harlot's door. That little nugget of time where you're struggling between options. Temptation isn't tangible reality. It exists entirely in your head.

Thus, eliminating temptation is an incredibly simple, one-step process. Decide beforehand what you will and will not do. Then, when a situation comes up, don't waver, waffle or debate. Just move into what you've already decided to do, on autopilot.

If this is how you handle challenges, you won't be bothered by temptations. There is no pause where you're struggling with your decision, so temptation won't exist for you! Live consciously. Don't let yourself be swayed each time the possibility for a poor choice comes up.

There may be times when you choose to indulge, that's true. But if you're doing it right, you will have made that decision beforehand. Eliminates guilt, too. Because guilt just sucks if you ask me.

Incidentally, a nice perk from this approach is that it completely disables potential saboteurs. If you clearly and decisively decline a bad choice immediately, there's no room for Mary the Meddler to elbow you in the side and nag, "Oh, just this once won't hurt you. C'mon! C'mon!"

Your "thanks but no thanks" has already been registered and you've moved on to more interesting things. Like where to find some of those veggies and dip!

When faced with a situation where your resolve may be tested, I realize we don't consciously plan through the string of thoughts and feelings that play out. But we do decide what to do with them, what we feed. And a long, tortured pause while we consider indulging is every bit as good as feeding the temptation. You're leaning against the harlot's door hard, man, and you're liable to fall in any second!

Forget the external situation. It doesn't matter anyway. Fact is, the responsibility is always yours. What are you doing? Are you hanging outside the harlot's door, mouth a-waterin'? Or do you briskly walk on by to wherever it is you really planned to go?

As LONG as you've decided you cannot pass temptation, you cannot. (And don't forget, you're risking a hard slap saying this around me.) But the point is, you make your own reality. Sorry, but you can't blame it on the cookie-wielding harlot.

You make the decision every day, every minute, who you want to be and how you want to handle life. And as they say in existentialism, life is a "prison of choices." Not making a choice is a choice in and of itself.

The responsibility always comes back home. And that is both disquieting and comforting at the same time.

See that harlot's door? Keep on walking, baby. Keep on walking!

CHAPTER 27

Motivation? Please, Girlfriend!

Ever heard chatter about people having trouble sticking to "the diet," not being motivated, yada, yada, yada?

Well, here's a fun fact for you. Motivation is NOT necessary to make changes. I repeat: motivation is not necessary to make changes. Heresy? Hear me out.

Motivation = the drive to accomplish something. Sound about right?

There are some things, any way you slice 'em, are and always will be unpleasant. Cutting the lawn. Cleaning the oven. Breaking up. Changing a diaper. The drive is not going to be there to experience this unpleasantness.

How do unpleasant things get done? Well, we know they need to get done, we know there are consequences for them not getting done, so we just get off our posteriors and do them. And after, we feel good because we've accomplished something.

Add to the no-motivation list: severely changing your lifestyle. Especially if, like me, you considered chocolate one of the basic food groups. Toward the bottom of my personal food pyramid.

So let's face it directly. This is no fun! Breaking old habits, leaving previous sources of comfort, dealing with the sometimes painful task of honestly facing up? Well, holy moly, man. That sucks! But it's worth it.

I guess you could name it "motivation" when you see the scale is careening wildly towards the upper end of capacity, or you almost mistake yourself in a picture for a VW bus.

I would offer another explanation. This is not motivation. It's pain. Embarrassment, fear, sadness, and all those associated feelings you get when you first acknowledge your weight is out of control? That is pain.

As is human nature, we seek to enhance pleasure and avoid pain. Survival 101. So what you see when people commit to losing the weight, that's nothing short of evolution in action. Hooray for evolution!

However, once you buck up and start making changes, motivation begins coming into play. You see progress. You see work paying off! You get the additional energy, you feel great, you look great, and you are great! And you like it. You want more, no?

So get this: motivation doesn't precede progress. Motivation follows and enhances progress. It maintains it and spurs it along once you start rolling.

But if you sit passively on your butt waiting to become properly motivated? Uh. Might as well start mainlining the chocolate syrup now, baby. 'Cause you ain't getting nowhere that way!

Every day, make choices that are more in line with your long-term goals than not. And the next thing you know, you're halfway there, man! Maybe it was a realization that started everything. Maybe it was pain. Maybe it was a shift in priorities that started you thinking a different way. But it's always the decision to change that precedes the change.

If you take full responsibility for what you've done with the body that you have, you give yourself a tremendous gift: the ability to change! Once you put it squarely within your control, you can fix it.

And that, my friends, is a treasure beyond value!

CHAPTER 28

Self-Definitions and Weight Loss

"The words 'I am...' are potent words; be careful what you hitch them to. The thing you're claiming has a way of reaching back and claiming you."
-A. L. Kitselman

You decide who you are by...well, deciding who you are. You know?

If you want to lose weight, but you say, "I'm too lazy to exercise; I'm too weak to pass up the cake; I have no willpower; I can't avoid temptation..." and such, you're going nowhere! Fact is, defining yourself as a failure doesn't make you successful. It just makes you fat.

You create reality with your self-definition. The principal applies for everything, by the way.

If you want to be more organized, for goodness sakes, don't sit around telling me what a disorganized mess you are! I don't give a fig about your reasons. First of all, focus on area you ARE doing well with organizing, and then, expand it. And all the while, tell yourself you're the epitome of organization, okay? That is what you need to do.

I can tell you this: if you tell yourself you can't do it, you won't. If you tell yourself you can do it, or even better, you ARE doing it, even if you don't believe 100% at first, you will believe it. Because it will start happening. Your words and perceptions will conspire to recreate your reality.

The thing that gets me is that people do this incessantly! Every time they want to make a change, they spend about half their energy explaining why they cannot possibly make the change, why they haven't made the change thus far, how much of a handicap they have in trying to make the change—all for reasons they firmly place as "beyond their control," on and on and on. The focus is 99% on shortcomings, faults, problems, stumbling blocks, you-name-it, whatever stops them from completing the job. They self-define as the opposite of what they say they hope to be.

You know what that tells me? If that's where your energy goes, complaining about how you cannot do whatever, defining yourself as someone incapable of making those changes, then deep down, you aren't ready. No matter how you may protest the factuality of this point. 'Cause if you were ready for the change, you wouldn't be sitting here telling me it is impossible to change.

You want to accomplish something big? Honestly? Then you have to begin by deciding it's at least a POSSIBILITY, for goodness sakes! Otherwise, why are you wasting everyone's time? You don't have to be totally on-board that it will all go fine and dandy.

At least, not yet. But you do have to see it as, at minimum, an option!

Then, you start focusing on what you're now doing, not why you haven't done it yet. Frankly, I have no interest in discussing why you haven't reached your goals. That's boring! Nine times out of ten, we're talking about a long list of half-assed excuses anyway. At least, that's what I produce when I climb into the poor-little-me mindset.

I'll tell you a little secret. If you move to exclusively focus on what you want and actively visualize yourself as reaching your goal, see yourself already there in the future reality, focusing on your strengths only, roadblocks magically begin to dissipate and just as magically, avenues for your success start showing up left and right. Yes, you'll still have to do whatever work you need to do, but what you'll find is that doors, ideas, support, and resources to help you will begin appearing out of thin air.

You think some people are just lucky? That opportunities show up for them at exactly the right time? Their luck comes from the energy they put out, the possibilities they open themselves up to seeing, and that energy is what draws what they need.

But don't just take my word for it. Try it, for a week. Pick your goal, whatever it is, end any negative talk about it completely, and replace it with language, thoughts and images of yourself currently being successful with your efforts. Make sure you acknowledge current progress and stuff you've already accomplished, too!

You don't have to have completely master it all to be successful. Progressing is just as vital as reaching the end. Without the progress, you'd never make it to the end, right?

Success isn't about the goal; it's about the journey, my friend! So get moving.

CHAPTER 29

What's Your Hurry, Sparky?

People get weird sometimes going on about how they DESERVE to lose weight but it hasn't happened. It almost seems like they're completely hacked off sometimes.

"Hey, I only ate 3 lettuce leaves and some chicken broth but I gained half a pound yesterday! Whyyyyyyy?"

Well, maybe because your body does not work like an accounting ledger where, if you put X in this column, then you get Y in that other column.

You are a biological organism. That means your body has an inherent degree of unpredictability. Don't like it? Well, try to find somebody to transplant your brain into a robot body, then, 'cause that's part of the human experience.

And while we're at it, I HATE it when somebody takes on a challenging tone with one of the "why ain't I losing?" quizzes. As if it's my job to make sure you lose to prove that my eating habits work. That's just annoying, man. Everybody is different and we all have to solve this puzzle ourselves. Get the chip off your shoulder, 'cause we're all just trying to help one another through this together.

And hey, it's not like you were sitting there griping and moaning the day you ate half a package of cookies and didn't gain weight, right? So why are you whining now? Get over it already. (I can get by with saying this, because I have done the same thing. Ha!)

It's completely NORMAL for your weight to fluctuate up to several pounds in a single DAY. Yep. In a single day! So if you're out there living and dying by the readout on your digital scale, you're gonna have some unnecessary pain, man.

The scale obsession seems to go hand-in-hand with, "How many minutes is it gonna take for me to lose this 50 pounds?" Sometimes followed up with "Because I'm going nuts here and I have my high school reunion in three hours and I'm getting married next week..."

Now, it's not like I don't get it. Oh boy, do I! I'll let you in on a little secret. The reason I can nail your butt on all these little sneaky thought-processes is that I've SO been there, too. I know because I did it. Can't get much by me.

I'm going to say something kind of radical here. I don't give a %$#% how quickly you lose it. And you shouldn't either.

If you want this to WORK, if you want to keep your weight OFF forever, you will need to adjust your eating habits forever. Start eating like you used to, you'll weigh what you used to.

So, can you see that it's actually better if it goes gradually? If it's all about speed, then it's not about lifetime habits.

Speed obsession = counting the minutes until you lose the weight–and, by implication, until you can "stop the diet."

So that really means counting the minutes until you start packing the pounds back on. Doesn't sound so good that way, does it?

TAKE YOUR TIME. It's not how fast you do it, it's how permanently you do it!

Almost everything in life seems to work better if you let go of the anxiety, the second-guessing, and the angst. Just let go and do your thing, man. That's where you find your Zen.

Once you get Zen, the rest starts to come much more naturally. That's definitely worth waiting for!

CHAPTER 30

Fat Thinking

I watch people. In particular, I watch folks with weight issues. And you can see certain attitudes, opinions, and self-stories that have a pretty strong correlation with failure rates.

Now, I'm not saying I don't think you can overcome dysfunctional attitudes. You certainly can. And they don't have any huge meaning, except in most cases, you'll be stuck until you move past them. If you spot yourself in here, don't take it too hard. I couldn't understand this all so well unless I'd had some degree of personal experience with many of these attitudes. (Most? All? I'll never tell!)

Fat Attitudes

"I just can't stick with this."

Granted, most everybody who struggles with weight has said this or something like it at one time or another. And often, it's simply a complaint, fussing at oneself for off-plan eating. But let's stop and take a closer look...

Here's what I say: As long as you're sitting there TELLING me you can't, I'm not going to argue with you about it. But the opposite is also true: you tell me you CAN, and it's true as well. So you can turn this around at any point.

But it's still not a good idea to say this. Because each time you say this, it sinks into your brain. Each time you say this, it becomes just a little more true. It becomes a little bit more real for you.

Instead, how about saying, "I feel frustrated because I haven't stuck with my eating plan?" Or better, use the words "haven't chosen" in the sentence. It IS a choice. Don't even pretend otherwise-at least, not around me. There are no cookie-wielding terrorists force-feeding you Oreos.

"I don't know what's wrong with me."

That one is easy: nothing! To say something is wrong with you implies that you have some sort of hidden defect that preempts your ability to lose weight. It's not your choices. It's that darn secret, inner defect! You know. The one that makes it so you can't stay on track more than 24 hours in a row...yeah! That one.

Now, you tell me that you don't understand why you're making choices that don't support your long-term goals, and I can buy that. But declaring yourself inherently defective is not only inaccurate, it's counter-productive. It keeps you from honestly examining why you are making non-helpful choices. It takes the power out of your hands and puts it off to the winds of fate. Screw that. Taking responsibility can sting a little bit, but it's the only way you can change.

"Ooopsie! I messed up and ate 2 dozen donuts and 4 big Macs. Twenty-two times. Heh heh. But I'll restart in 253 days on January 1st."

Well, heck. Number one, it's not cute when you sabotage yourself. Period. I mean, sure, it's fine and good to laugh at yourself about a lot of things. Most things, really. But still. It's just not cute to mess up and keep messing up.

And number two, WHY on earth would you want to wait to get back on track? You need MORE to overcome before you get back on track? This makes so little sense it makes my hair hurt.

It doesn't matter if it's in the morning or Monday or next week or January 1st. Your behind doesn't fail to pack on pounds just because you think you should be able to live consequence-free on the weekends. The butt cannot read a calendar.

"I have to do it this time. There is no choice. It's my last chance."

This one doesn't sound so bad, does it? Adding that extra motivation to get it right? See, it's still dysfunctional in my opinion.

Why? Well, because it's not true for starters! You're not going to blow your brains out if you don't lose twelve pounds by next Friday, right? (It has to be by Friday, 'cause you know...your backside won't let you lose weight on a weekend.)

You'd better realize there IS a choice. 'Cause if you're not acknowledging a choice, once again your signing off your personal power to the wind— or the Chinese buffet. And that will get you nowhere.

And if you've touted this as the absolute last chance, what happens if it doesn't go as planned? You give up?

How about this—your "last chance" is when you quit, plain and simple. You don't fail until you quit forever. And if you've quit a thousand times, then you damn well better restart 1001 times. If you actually want to be successful, that is.

"They made me eat that cake."

Give me a break, man. If there are no firearms involved, nobody made you eat squat. And your butt doesn't care who told you to eat it. There is a special, magical spell that you can use in this situation. You utter the magic word as many times as it takes—one more time than they demand you eat—and it all goes away. They word is "No." Yeah, I know you knew that.

I have to have the [insert Junk Food Item] for my husband/kids/mother/imaginary friend.

I mean, you know this is baloney even when you're saying it, don't you? Who's gonna die without their snack cakes? And if your family relationships are going to fall apart without full and unrestricted toaster pastry access, if some sugar-squares are more important to your family than your health and well-being...well, geez. I'm at a loss for words on that. In that case, you have some problems I cannot really help with. Family might moan and whine to start, but from what I've seen, in the long run they'll get over it.

Now, I poke fun at these attitudes. Because really, we need to see the silliness. We need to see it's ridiculous so we can quit thinking this way.

See, you're very possibly reading this as someone who's been struggling with your weight, maybe for a long time. And each of the other times, maybe you've had these attitudes or similar. They don't serve you. So cut 'em out.

Just take care of today, focus on the process, focus on now, and drop the excuses. And the future has an amazing way of taking care of itself. If you take care of right this minute, man. Even if it's Saturday night. Your butt will thank you.

Now just shut up and do it.

CHAPTER 31

Why Won't They Listen?

"I feel great, but I can't get my [insert-person-you-love-here] to make the healthy changes I'm making, even though they really need to. Their health is at stake! Why can't they understand, and how can I make them understand how important this is?"

This is a familiar refrain from people who've made changes to their eating habits, lost weight, and are enthusiastic about their progress. You feel great, you look great, and you are great! It's natural to want to share this awesomeness with others you care about. You want them to feel better and become healthier too. You worry about them, after all. You want only what's best for them, and they know that. You try and try to convince them, but to no avail.

So why won't they listen? And more importantly, what can you do about it?

Take a trip back in time now. Think of yourself, before you embarked on your quest. Whether you were happy or not most of the time yourself, it's almost certain there were others in your life that weren't. Were there at least occasions when somebody was trying to convince you to lose some of the flab? It could have been anybody, from your doctor to your 3-year-old. Just take a second and remember...how did you feel about it?

Did the nagging, exhortations, dire warnings, or anything else coming at you make ANY difference at all?

For me, it made a difference all right. Being told I wasn't okay just how I was made me even more determined to stay exactly as I was! It had the exact opposite effect from the intentions, however well-meaning. "Screw 'em!" That's how I felt. Like me as I am, or I don't need you.

Criticism, however constructive it's intended. just doesn't work well for most people. And nobody probably could have pushed you into losing the weight one flat second before you were ready to do so yourself, right? I mean, okay. For real, lasting and significant changes, the desire for change has to come from within.

So where does that leave you? How can you make them see the light?

Short answer? You don't. Nobody makes anybody else see the light. People see whatever light they are ready to see, whenever they are ready to see it and not a millisecond sooner.

But you can help, and help a lot! It's just not the nagging, whiney, cajoling sort of help most people try. It's a million times easier, and more pleasant for everybody.

You help others see and share your success by living it. You back off from the pushing and pulling.

You make your own decisions, and allow your loved ones to make their own decisions.

When your decisions are working for you (and working very well, thank you), you radiate the strong, positive energy that comes from being in a good place. You don't have to try and convince people that if they change their ways they can have what you've got. They can see it! You don't have to try and sell them the potential benefits that comes from being kind to their bodies. You're a walking billboard for making positive changes. You wear it every day.

This holds true of the "no support at home" issue as well. Maybe your spouse is tired of seeing you frustrated with yourself and disappointed on yet another weight loss plan. Or maybe s/he is just a bit insecure, and is worried you will be out the door if you slim down too much. Maybe your kids don't want to give up your delicious cookies, or resent the ever-present supply line of snack cakes has dried up. I don't know.

But it doesn't matter much, because people who care about you want to see you happy in the long run. They'll get over their issues. Your best argument for making healthy changes—be it for yourself or others—is ALWAYS demonstrating the positive outcome of those changes.

So, ultimately: If you want to help others around you to share some of the success you're having, there is one very powerful way to do that. Be highly successful! Your example is much more powerful than your arguments (which most overweight people are intimately familiar with already). Your example is more powerful than your dire health warnings (which most overweight people have already tuned out years ago).

One of the main differences is that your positive example comes from a place that feels good. There's no implied criticism, control issues, warnings of horrendous outcomes, or negative energy of any kind attached to your success. It becomes easier for others to attach to that which feels good.

Of course, you may well be asking yourself, "Well, what if they still don't decide to lose the weight, despite my good example?" That's entirely possible. They may not, now. They may not, possibly ever. They may decide to do whatever the heck they want, whenever the heck they want to, forever more. What then?

What then? A big, fat, nothing. You love 'em exactly the way they are, as long as they choose to stay that way.

We get so invested in other people's choices sometimes that we lose sight of the larger picture. Regardless of the relationship, we sometimes see their choices as vital to our own health, happiness and well-being. That's a very unstable place to be, let me tell ya. Whoo doggie!

Yes, there's no question: if you're connected to others, their choices impact you. Well, duh! But the point is, everyone's life belongs to them. Everyone's health is their own, to care for or disregard, as they see fit. Even your spouse, or your kids or your mother-in-law's cousin: everyone owns their own life. As you own your own life.

It is not an emergency if people you care about make choices you don't agree with! It can sure feel like a catastrophe, I know. I have grown kids. I have therefore seen people I care about with every cell of my body make choices that I know may have dire, even life-threatening consequences. Literally. And continue and continue and continue to make choices that I perceive as highly dangerous and destructive. And you know what I could do about it? Not much, man.

One thing I learned from parenting: the harder you push someone, the harder they push back. You can be objectively right and they can even know it, but it makes no difference.

Instead of conceding, they become more and more entrenched and it becomes an issue of pride at some point. There's no way to back down without losing face. Nobody likes to feel stupid and humiliated on top of acknowledging they have to make serious changes, too. Or maybe they just tune you out and go on. Whatever is happening in their head, it is all too clear that the strong-arm pressure techniques don't do squat.

But oddly enough, you never can know that anyone else is actually wrong. I don't really care what it's about. I spent many years overweight. That doesn't mean that was wrong. In fact, I think the experience taught me tons! (Ha, ha! I said "tons.")

Much of what I learned then, I now use to help others. I became more sensitive in many ways. I have been able to use that experience to become, I believe, a better person. So who's to say I was wrong?

You make the choices you make based on where you're at and what you need to learn. That's how you end up in these situations to begin with. It's true that some choices lead to pleasure, and some to pain. But even those choices leading to pain serve a vital function: learning. Always, always, there is learning to be had. If you fight the lessons, they come back harder and stronger. But then again, the lessons wouldn't be coming unless you needed them, pretty much by definition.

Pain serves a tremendously important function, In psych class many years ago, I learned about people who, because of a rare medical condition, don't feel pain at all. Nothing! At first blush, this sounds like a tremendous boon, right? Who wouldn't like to have a life free of any physical pain? Sounds great!

Most of these people, however, had very short lives. Without pain to warn them of danger, they had no impetus for escaping. They couldn't tell when they were being hurt. They literally "didn't know what hit them."

Sometimes, people simply need to be shaken up to reach saturation level with the status quo. Crisis often leads to turning points. I know you'd prefer not to see those you love go through the crisis to begin with. Of course not! But really, the most loving thing you can do is give those around you enough room to do their own work.

You're not doing anyone any favors by trying to spare them their lessons, regardless of the intent. You don't spare them anything, and damage your own relationship with them in the process.

Bottom line: if someone you care for isn't making the choices you'd like them to, well...it's simply none of your business.

Your business is to stand tall, strong, and serve as an example of all the benefits of taking care of yourself. Love others enough to give them room to learn their own lessons. They will learn what they need to, when they're darned good and ready and not a moment before.

Just like you.

Peace out to you, and yours.

CHAPTER 32

Self-Esteem: Chicken or Egg?

Answer this as True or False: "After I lose all this extra weight, I'll feel better about myself."

Did you agree? If so, I've got a surprise for you-it's not true! Losing weight does not make you feel better about yourself. Shocked? I was, too, when I realized this.

People often DO feel better about themselves after losing weight, but it's NOT the number on the scale that performs the wizardy. And in learning to differentiate, you can actually lose weight easier and be more likely to keep it off, not to mention become happier in the process.

When people work on their weight, there are two very distinct dimensions. There is the one we all pay attention to, the physical dimension. The physical is represented in clothing sizes, inches lost, and of course, the scale, a contrary little contraption that is our best friend or worst nemesis, depending on the day. It's the meal plans, the carb counts, the food logs and macro counts. It's the exercise and the sweat. It's all those things most typically associate with dieting.

What most people ignore, however, it the mental dimension. The mental dimension is expressed in the body image you have in your head, plus your beliefs about yourself, your sense of power, strength, worthiness and self-love (or self-hate). This is what you believe about yourself, your wants and desires, and your drive for growth. This is where potential is born.

You wonder why so many people can lose weight but don't keep it off? It's because they only master the physical! Addressing the physical dimension of weight loss isolated from the mental dimension is like running hip-deep in water against the current to reach a goal. You can get there, but it becomes a struggle to make each little bit of progress. As soon as you let up and fight it less, the current starts to sweep you backwards. And even when you get to your destination, you still have to expend considerable energy to stay still.

The oft-neglected mental dimension, however, is what directs the current. It addresses momentum. It's what brings the energy into motion and determines the rate and strength of said motion.

And I'm here to tell you that if you master the mental adjustments, the physical will fall into place more or less effortlessly. It will become EASY.

In other words, you don't feel better about yourself after you lose weight. You lose weight after you start feeling better about yourself!

This is a big one, so take a minute to let it sink in.

While you may think that this is all over-simplistic metaphysical hoohaw, it's absolutely true. Think for a minute. You know anyone who is financially comfortable who thinks, speaks, visualizes or even actively hates poverty? You know anyone who is healthy who thinks, speaks, visualizes or actively hates illness? You know anyone who is happy who thinks, speaks, visualizes or actively hates sadness?

You don't become thin by thinking about fatness, speaking about fatness, visualizing fatness or hating your fat! In fact, hatred is a very concentrated form of energy. The mind-body connection is well-documented at this point, but not well understood. However, it's not necessary to understand the mechanism to use it to your advantage.

To be successful, focus on success. Any success will do, be it yours, someone else's, weight-related, or not. You surround yourself with positive, uplifting feelings. You constantly build yourself up, up, up. Success breeds more success.

To put it simply, to be, to do or have anything at all, you have to start moving your energy in that direction.

While you can do this with oppressive dieting, harsh workout routines and utter self-disgust, that isn't the most comfortable (or lasting) way to go about it. That's trying to walk against the current. Not only does an oppressive, self-denigrating approach feel terrible, it doesn't stick. Sooner or later, you will "backslide" into a stance that doesn't leave you hating yourself. Small wonder, huh?

A much happier (and easier) way of moving your energy in the direction you want to go is taking small steps bringing you closer to your goals, and most important of all, feel GOOD about them.

The steps you take needn't be painful. In fact, they shouldn't be! A little of this, and a little more, you think. A little of that, and a little more, you do. You listen to your body, your inner guidance, and trust yourself to make appropriate decisions. You find yourself feeling out the direction of the current, and riding it.

And the whole time, keep tuning in. Do you feel GOOD about the changes you're making? Do you feel stronger, happier, healthier, and more in control? Do you feel like you like where you're at more and more all the time? That means you're doing it right!

Don't focus on any perceived deficiencies. Focus solely on accomplishments! If you feel good about your choices, that means you're almost certainly moving in the right direction.

The better you feel about yourself, the simpler it is to lose weight. Personally, I suspect that feeling healthier creates a sort of biofeedback loop that speeds up your metabolism or something. I can't exactly explain it, but I don't care. It works.

I have seen many people gain and lose weight over and over again. The ones that lose and keep it off are the ones that have intact self-images (which, incidentally, seem to bear no correlation to their starting size).

And it makes sense, too. Happy people don't need to adjust mood via sugar-therapy.

It's hard to stay focused on your goals when you feel undeserving, by virtue of not having reached the goals yet. Huh? But that's what people so often do.

And worse, even when you reach your goals, if you feel, deep down, the success is not deserved, you will find ways to subconsciously undo all the work you just did.

If you don't change what's in your brain, any changes in your body are temporary at best. Your brain will always bring you back around to what you secretly believe defines you.

When you lose weight after deciding to do so, it is motivating and reinforcing. Absolutely! But that sense of feeling better about yourself is more about feeling in control, feeling your own power, than it is about a smaller pants size. It's about recognizing and acknowledging your worth. It's about pride in making healthy changes and following through.

Believe me, there are plenty of skinny people who hate themselves, and plenty of fat people who love themselves. So get that whole "losing the belly will solve all my problems" crap right out of your head.

If you want to materialize a thinner body, better health, more energy, more or better anything, then you have to tune in to that frequency. You focus on it, daydream about how great it will feel, enjoy your progress in the direction you're going, celebrating victories each step of the way. You surround yourself with positive thoughts and feelings, and then? You attune to it. Then you can just hop into the current and achieve it with Zen intact.

It's fine to like yourself, too, no matter what you weigh. If you take nothing else from this book, take that thought and make it your own. I promise you, it will make a tremendous, positive impact in your life.

♥ YOU ARE GOOD ENOUGH ALREADY! ♥

Epilogue: What Now?

These words have been sitting in files on my computer for literally years. I originally wrote the early drafts of this material when I led (the now-defunct) Low Carb Eating and Shrinking Goddess weight loss support sites.

I was neck deep in my own weight loss journey and trying very hard to help folks address the issues that I saw cropping up again and again and again—many of which I had experienced personally. At the time, I was totally rocking it, a stellar example of low carb success story.

I still consider myself a success story. But it's not been without significant detours.

While I never abandoned low carb completely (nor will I), truth is that I was no longer the very clearly successful low carber I once was. I could give you a list of reasons why, but nobody cares—including me! Part of the reason I moved on from those roles was the staggering responsibility of being looked to as an example when many times, I felt totally unsuited for the task. I still do, if you want to know the absolute, God's-honest truth.

I was trying, very hard, I might add, to retire from the low carb spotlight when I ended up with another successful low carb community quite by accident. Suffice it to say, nobody was more shocked than me when my little public service, low carb Facebook page—the one I didn't have the heart to delete—went viral through the help of some smart friends. So I came back to the Low Carb world with a bang, sporting a quickly growing audience and dazed expression.

Now, I am healthy and I feel good. While I'm perfectly okay with where I am, I realize some people judge a weight loss writer by pants size and mine remains in the double digits.

Believe me, I'm well aware at how harsh people can be about folks in the weight loss community who are not perceived as appropriately lean—even among those who should know better. So even putting myself out here this much makes me a target for criticism.

But that's okay. I can weather whatever is hurled at me. You know why?

Because I get email after email from our fans. They tell me we do at Low Carb Zen MATTERS.

People have gotten off medications, reversed the progress of diabetes and high blood pressure, lost weight, sure, but so much more! It changes people's lives, changing how they eat.

Your emails have brought me to tears more times that I can count. I am moved by your stories and enormously grateful I've gotten to play even a small part in your journey. I'm humbled beyond belief and stupidly grateful for the chance to make a real difference in people's lives.

So that's why I share recipes day after day. That's why I answer the very same questions over and over. That's why I post my own dumb casserole recipes with crappy pictures, even though I'm about as ill-qualified to be a food blogger as anyone you'll ever find. That's why I make videos (even if some people think I'm too fat) and that's why I keep preaching the gospel about being kind to your body and eating healthy food.

Because it MATTERS. For me and for you.

But all of this is for naught if you don't walk the path, you know? So do me a favor.

I don't care where you are at. It doesn't matter if you have 4 pounds to lose or 400. It doesn't matter if you make big changes or little ones.

Just here and now, change SOMETHING for the better. Today. Right now. One little step, because each step counts. And I'll make a deal with you: I'll do the same. Fair enough?

If I've helped encourage you to make a single change for the better, my work here has been a success. So make me a success, please! And if you want to tell me about it, shoot me an email at dix@lowcarbzen.com. I'll be cheering you on.

Much love & Peace Out.
~Dix

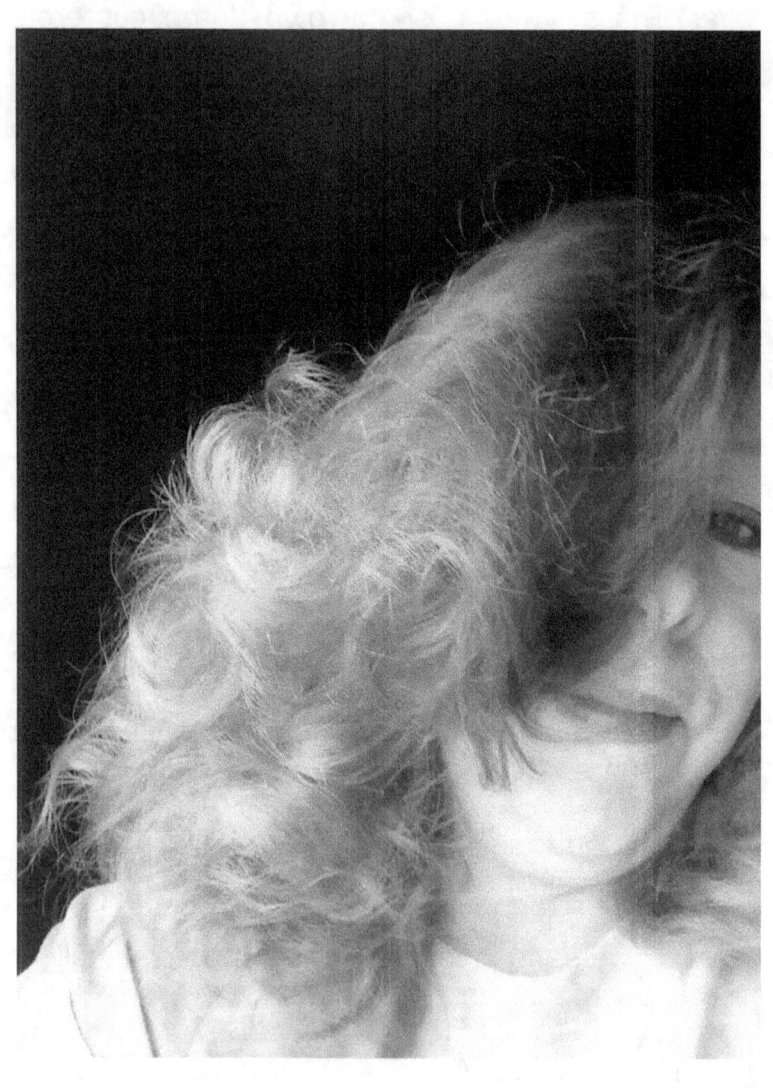

About The Author

Dixie Vogel is still more than a little stunned she can un-ironically add "food blogger" to her resume. She usually describes herself as a "Pink-Haired Hippie Chick & Eccentric Genius."

Although lately, she's taken to referring to herself as "the World's Unlikeliest Food Blogger" because she's doing it, but ain't a fancypants chef-type by any stretch.

In fact, this whole "low carb empire" thing just kind of happened while she was busy not trying. Her kitchen stubbornly remains an a mess and she boasts no outrageously adorable toddlers to exploit as recipe photo props. (Somehow, Thor the Warrior Kitten licking a beater does not hold the same appeal. And besides, he just keeps wiggling out of those darned aprons.)

But Dixie does understand the psychology of weight loss intimately, spending most of her life significantly overweight before losing over a hundred pounds. She considers herself just your average chick who use to be a whole lot heavier but now isn't, thanks to the magic of low carb.

In the process of finding her own weight loss Zen, Dixie has been fortunate enough to touch millions through leading weight loss support communities, culminating with the current and most popular, Low Carb Zen (https://www.lowcarbzen.com).

Dixie also slings Tarot, teaches the mystical arts and offers one-on-one consultations and coaching at A Fool's Journey (http://www.afoolsjourney.com).

Dixie lives in Kansas with her husband of a quarter century plus, and some criminally spoiled cats. And there are all those birds, who seem to follow her wherever she goes.

She likes those birds. They talk to her.

www.ingramcontent.com/pod-product-compliance
Lightning Source LLC
Chambersburg PA
CBHW071353280526
45787CB00001B/307